THE ULTIMATE
SURVIVAL
MEDICINE
GUIDE
EMERGENCY PREPAREDNESS FOR ANY DISASTER

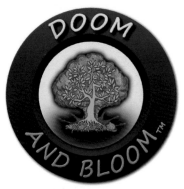

JOSEPH ALTON, MD
AMY ALTON, ARNP

Skyhorse Publishing

DISCLAIMER

The information given and opinions voiced in this volume are for educational and entertainment purposes only and do not constitute medical advice or the practice of medicine. No provider-patient relationship, explicit or implied, exists among the publisher, authors, and readers. This book does not substitute for such a relationship with a qualified provider. As many of the strategies discussed in this volume would be less effective than proven present-day medications and technology, the authors and publisher strongly urge their readers to seek modern and standard medical care with certified practitioners whenever and wherever it is available.

The reader should never delay seeking medical advice, disregard medical advice, or discontinue medical treatment because of information in this book or any resources cited in this book.

Although the authors have researched all sources to ensure accuracy and completeness, they assume no responsibility for errors, omissions, or other inconsistencies therein. Neither do the authors or publisher assume liability for any harm caused by the use or misuse of any methods, products, instructions, or other information in this book or any resources cited in this book.

Skyhorse Publishing books may be purchased in bulk at special discounts for sales promotion, corporate gifts, fund-raising, or educational purposes. Special editions can also be created to specifications. For details, contact the Special Sales Department, Skyhorse Publishing, 307 West 36th Street, 11th Floor, New York, NY 10018 or info@skyhorsepublishing.com.

Skyhorse® and Skyhorse Publishing® are registered trademarks of Skyhorse Publishing, Inc.®, a Delaware corporation.

Visit our website at www.skyhorsepublishing.com.

15

Library of Congress Cataloging-in-Publication Data is available on file.

Cover design by Brian Peterson
Cover photo credit: Thinkstockphotos.com
ISBN: 978-1-62914-770-3
Ebook ISBN: 978-1-63220-261-1

Printed in China

This book is dedicated to my wife, Amy, the person who first made it clear to me that this book was needed by those who want to be medically prepared in times of trouble.

—Joseph Alton, MD

I dedicate this book to my husband, Joe, a man dedicated to his mission: to put a medically prepared person in every family for any disaster.

—Amy Alton, ARNP

In addition, we both dedicate this book to those who are ready to serve as medical resources in times of disaster. We salute your courage in accepting this assignment; have no doubt, you will save lives.

—Joseph Alton, MD, and Amy Alton, ARNP

"Do what you can, with what you have, where you are."

—Theodore Roosevelt

ABOUT THE AUTHORS

Joseph Alton practiced as a board-certified obstetrician and pelvic surgeon for more than twenty-five years before retiring to devote his efforts to preparing families medically for any scenario. He is a fellow of the American College of Obstetrics and Gynecology and the American College of Surgeons, and served as department chairman at local hospitals and as an adjunct professor at local university nursing schools. He is a contributor to well-known preparedness magazines and is frequently invited to speak at survival and preparedness conferences throughout the country. A member of MENSA, Dr. Alton collects medical books from the nineteenth century to gain insight on off-the-grid medical protocols.

Amy Alton is an advanced registered nurse practitioner and a certified nurse-midwife. She has had years of experience working in large teaching institutions as well as smaller, family-oriented hospitals. Amy has extensive medicinal herb and vegetable gardens and works to include natural remedies into her gardening strategies.

As "Dr. Bones and Nurse Amy," these medical professionals host a medical preparedness website at www.doomandbloom.net and produce video and radio programs under the Doom and Bloom™ label. Dr. and Ms. Alton are firm believers that, to remain healthy in hard times, we must use all the tools in the medical woodshed. Their goal is to promote integrated medicine; in this way, they can offer their readers the most options to keep their loved ones healthy in a long-term survival situation.

TABLE OF CONTENTS

+++

INTRODUCTION

✚ ✚ ✚

Most outdoor medicine guides are intended to aid you in managing emergency situations in austere and remote locations. Certainly, modern medical care on an ocean voyage or wilderness hike is not readily available; even trips to cities in underdeveloped countries may fit this category. Despite this, we all expect that the rescue helicopter is on the way.

What is your goal when an emergency occurs in a remote setting? The basic premise of emergency medicine in the field is to

- ☤ Evaluate the injured or ill patient.
- ☤ Stabilize their condition.
- ☤ Transport them to the nearest modern medical facility.

This series of steps makes perfect sense: you are not a physician and there are facilities that have a lot more technology than you have in your backpack. Your priority is to get the patient out of immediate danger and to a hospital. Transporting the injured person may be difficult to do (sometimes very difficult), but you still have the luxury of being able to "pass the buck" to those who have more knowledge, technology, and supplies.

This is a perfectly reasonable approach. One day, however, there may come a time when a pandemic, civil unrest, or a terrorist event may precipitate a situation where the miracle of modern medicine may be unavailable—indeed, not only unavailable, but even to the point that the potential for access to modern facilities no longer exists.

We refer to this type of long-term scenario as a "collapse." In a collapse, you will have more risk for illness and injury than on a hike in the woods, yet little or no hope of obtaining more advanced care than you, yourself, can provide. Help is not on the way; therefore, *you* have become the place where the "buck" stops for the foreseeable future.

Few people are willing to even entertain the possibility that such a tremendous burden might be placed upon them. Even for those stalwarts who are willing, there are few books that will consider this drastic turn of events. Yet the likelihood of such a situation, over a lifetime, may not be so small.

Almost all guides on wilderness or developing-world medicine usually end with "Go to the hospital immediately." Although this is excellent advice where and when hospitals are available and functioning normally, it won't be very helpful in an extreme event, where the hospitals might be out of commission. We only have to look at Hurricane Katrina in 2005 to know that even modern medical facilities may be useless if they are understaffed, undersupplied, and overcrowded.

Disaster medical-assistance teams are overwhelmed when thousands need help at once, as in Katrina. Each household becomes the end of the line when it comes to its own well-being. In this circumstance, individuals and families must accumulate medical supplies to deal with varied emergencies on their own. Medical knowledge must be obtained and shared.

These medical supplies and skills must then be adjusted to fit a new mindset: that things have changed, perhaps for the long term, and that you are the best medical asset your family has.

Many will decide that they cannot bear the burden of being in charge of the medical care of other people. Others, however, will find the fortitude to grit their teeth and wear the badge of survival "medic." These individuals may have some medical experience, but most will simply be fathers and mothers, or other responsible adults, who understand that someone must be appointed to handle things when medical help is not forthcoming.

If this reality first becomes apparent when a loved one becomes ill or injured, the likelihood that you will have the training and supplies needed to be an effective medical provider will be close to zero. This is a sure way to ensure that, when everything else fails, you will, too.

This book is meant to educate and prepare those who want to ensure the health of their loved ones. If you can absorb the information here, you will be better equipped to handle 90 percent of the emergencies that you would see in a power-down scenario, whether after a societal collapse or after a more typical disaster scenario. You will also have a realistic view of what medical issues are survivable without modern facilities. We hope to give you the tools to arrive at choices that will increase your chances of successfully treating injuries and disease.

All the information in this book is meant for use in a postcollapse setting, when modern medicine is no longer available. If your leg is broken in five places, it stands to reason that you'll do better in an orthopedic hospital ward than with a splint made out of two sticks and strips from a T-shirt, if you have that option.

The strategies discussed here are not the most effective means of taking care of certain medical problems. In fact, some of them are straight out of the last century. They adhere to the philosophy that something is better than nothing; in a survival situation, that "something" might just get you through the storm. As Theodore Roosevelt once said, "You must do what you can, with what you have, where you are."

We hope that you'll never need to use the information in this book. Yet, disasters do happen and could tax even existing advanced medical systems. In that scenario, the information provided here will be valuable while you are waiting for help to arrive. With some medical knowledge and supplies, you may gain precious time for an injured loved one and aid in their recovery.

Keep in mind an important caveat: The practice of medicine or dentistry without a license is against the law. None of the recommendations in this book will protect you from liability when there is a functioning government and legal system. Consider obtaining formal medical education if you want to become a healthcare provider in a society that has not collapsed.

Although you will not be a physician after reading this book, you will certainly be more of a medical asset to your family, group, or community than you were before. Among other things, you will have

- Learned to think about what to do when you become the end of the line in terms of your family's medical well-being.
- Considered preventative medicine.
- Put together a medical kit for times of trouble.
- Thought about how to improvise in an austere setting.

Most importantly, you will have become medically prepared to face the uncertain future.

What This Book Isn't...

Although the information in this book will be useful to prepare for a major disaster or long-term catastrophe, it will not meet the needs of certain people. If you are already a doctor or formally trained medical professional, you may think you're already prepared and do not need the information in this book.

You would be right; this book is not primarily intended for you. It is meant for nonmedical professionals who are concerned about keeping their families healthy when trained personnel are unavailable.

This book might have some use, however, for the flexibly minded medical pro. In a long-term survival situation, medical personnel will not have the luxury to "stabilize and transport" and will have to adjust their mindset to fit the scenarios for which we wrote this book.

We also do not claim that this book is a comprehensive review of every topic covered in it. Don't expect, for example, fifty pages on how to treat athlete's foot.

This book is not meant for the person who expects to perform advanced medical procedures in the wilderness or any other power-down survival setting. You will not learn how to perform a cardiac bypass by reading this book, nor will you be learning how to reattach an amputated leg.

If nothing else, this book is realistic. It does not claim to cure problems that only modern technology will help. You will, however, be able to deal with the survivable issues you would encounter in an austere setting.

This book is about integrated medicine, so if you are dead set against either conventional or alternative methods of healing, you will not be happy with this book. This book looks at what is likely to be of benefit in emergency situations where supplies are limited. It aims to use *all* the tools in the medical woodshed. With it, you'll have the best chance of maintaining the long-term health of your family or community.

I.

✚ ✚ ✚

PRINCIPLES OF MEDICAL PREPAREDNESS

MEDICAL PREPAREDNESS: HOW TO GET STARTED

The focus of this book is medical preparedness: the ability to deal with sickness and injuries in tough times. Of course, anyone wishing to survive must first have food, water, and a shelter of some sort. A full stomach and protection from the elements will be the top priority. What, then, is next on the list?

After gathering food and building a shelter, many prepared individuals consider personal and home defense to be the most important priority in the event of a societal collapse. Certainly, defending oneself is important, but have you thought about defending your health?

In a situation where power might be down and normal methods of filtering water and cleaning food don't exist, your health is as much under attack as the survivors in the latest zombie apocalypse movie. Infectious diseases would likely become rampant, and it will be a challenge to maintain sanitary conditions. Simple activities of daily survival, such as chopping wood, commonly lead to cuts that could get infected. These minor issues, so easily treated by modern medical science, can easily become life threatening if left untreated in a disaster.

You may be an accomplished outdoorsman and have plenty of food and your share of defensive weaponry. Yet, what would you say to a member of your family who becomes ill or injured in a remote and austere setting? The difficulties involved in a grid-down situation will surely put the health of your entire family or group at risk. It's important to have training and supplies to deal with infections and injuries.

In a collapse, there will likely be a lot more diarrheal disease than gunfights at the O.K. corral. History teaches us that, in the Civil War, there were more deaths from dysentery than there were from bullet wounds.

If you make the commitment to learn how to treat medical issues and to store medical supplies properly, you're taking a genuine first step towards ensuring your family's survival in dark times. The medical supplies are more likely to be there if the unforeseen happens, and the knowledge you gain will be there for the rest of your life. Many medical supplies have long shelf lives; their longevity will be one of the factors that will give you confidence when moving forward. And let's not ignore their value as barter items in times of trouble.

We also encourage you to learn about natural remedies and alternative therapies that may have some benefit for different issues. We cannot vouch for the effectiveness of every claim that one thing or another will cure what ails you. Suffice it to say that our family has an extensive medicinal garden and that it might be a good idea for your family to have one, too. Many herbs that have medicinal properties are hardy and do well in less than optimal conditions for most plants, so a green thumb is not required to cultivate them. Many of them do not even require full sun to thrive.

It's important to understand that some illnesses will be difficult to treat if modern medical facilities aren't available. It will be hard to do much about those clogged coronary arteries—there won't be many cardiac bypasses performed. However, by ensuring good nutrition, you will give yourself the best chance to minimize some major medical issues. In a survival situation, an ounce of prevention is worth not a pound but a ton of cure. Start off healthy, and you'll have the best chance to stay that way.

We're not asking you to do anything that your great-grandparents didn't do as part of their strategy for succeeding in life. In a collapse, we'll be thrown back, in a way, to that era. It's important to learn some of the methods they used to stay healthy.

Some members of our family wonder why we spend all our time trying to prepare people medically for a major disaster. Despite history teaching us otherwise, they are totally certain that there is no scenario that would take away, even temporarily, the wonders of high technology. They tell me that we can't turn everyone into doctors, so why should we try?

Are we trying to turn everyone into doctors? No, there's too much to learn in one lifetime. Even as medical professionals, we often come across medical situations we're not sure about. That's what medical books are for, so make sure that you put together a survival library. You can refer to them when you need to, just as we do.

We are, however, trying to make you a better medical asset to your family and community than you were before. We firmly believe that, even if you have not undergone a formal medical education, you can learn how to treat the majority of problems you will encounter in a grid-down situation. You can, if necessary, be the end of the line with regards to the medical well-being of your people.

If you can absorb the information we provide in this guide, you will be in a position to help when the worst happens. Maybe, one day, you might even save a life; if that happens just once, our mission will have been a success.

WILDERNESS MEDICINE VS. LONG-TERM SURVIVAL MEDICINE

What is wilderness (also referred to as outdoor) medicine? We define it as medical care rendered in a situation where modern care, training, and facilities are not readily available. Wilderness medicine would involve medical care rendered during wilderness hikes, maritime expeditions, and sojourns in less-developed countries.

The basic assumption is that trained doctors and modern hospitals exist but are unavailable at the time that medical care is required (perhaps for a significant period of time). You, as temporary caregiver, will be responsible for stabilizing the patient. That means not allowing the injury or illness to get worse.

Your primary goal will be the evacuation of the patient to modern medical facilities, even though they might be hundreds of miles away from the location of the patient. Once you have transferred your patient to the next highest medical resource, your responsibility to the sick or injured individual will be over. Emergency medical technicians (EMTs) or military corpsmen will recognize this strategy as "stabilize and transport."

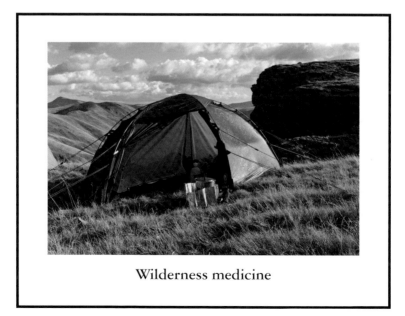

Wilderness medicine

Although principles of wilderness medicine have saved many lives, this approach is different from what we would call "long-term survival" or "collapse medicine." In a societal collapse, there is no access to modern medical care and no potential for such access in the foreseeable future.

As a result of this turn of events, you would go from being a temporary first-aid provider to being the caregiver at the end of the line. You become the highest medical resource left, regardless of whether you have a medical diploma.

This fact will lead you to make adjustments to your medical strategy. You are now responsible for the long-term care of the patient. As such, if you want to be successful in your new position, you will have to obtain more knowledge and training than you have now. You will also need more supplies if you intend to maintain the well-being of your family or friends. You will need a plan to deal with their potential medical needs.

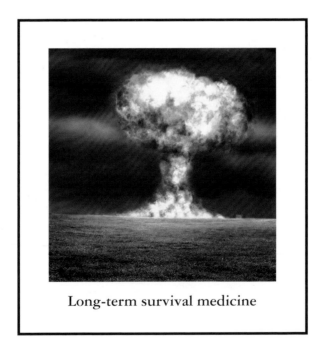

Long-term survival medicine

Medical training and education for nonphysicians can include wilderness medical classes, EMT, and even military medical corps training. These courses presuppose that you are rendering care in the hope of later transporting your patient to a working clinic, emergency room, or field hospital. If you can make the commitment, this training is very useful to have; it's much more likely that you'll experience a short-term deficit of medical assistance than a long-term one.

Despite this, you must plan for the possibility that you will be completely on your own one day. The way you think about this must be modified to fit a day when intensive care units and emergency rooms are inaccessible. You won't have the luxury of passing the sick or injured individual to a formally trained provider, so you must be ready to be there for your patient from start to finish.

You will also have to understand how to treat certain chronic medical conditions. Even a paramedic, for example, is unlikely to know how to deal with an abscessed tooth or a thyroid condition in the absence of drugs and high technology that may not be available.

Therefore, you must learn methods that will work in a power-down scenario; you may even have to reach back to older strategies that modern medicine might consider obsolete. Using a combination of prevention, improvisation, and prudent use of supplies, you should be able to treat the great majority of problems you will face in a power-down scenario.

Although all of this might seem daunting, we hope to impart enough information in this guide to make you confident in your new role. When you learn what to do in any scenario, you will feel that quiet resolve which comes with the knowledge that you can do the job. You'll be up to the challenge before you, and you'll know it.

THE IMPORTANCE OF COMMUNITY

Let's suppose that a calamity has occurred, and you have survived. The power grid is down, and is unlikely to be up again for years. You, however, have prudently stored food, medical sup-

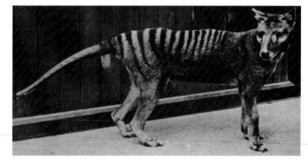

plies, and farming and hunting equipment and are safe in your shelter. You are a fine, young, strapping individual with no medical issues and are reasonably intelligent. Unfortunately, you haven't the slightest idea what the first thing is that you should do to ensure your future health and survival.

The very first way to help ensure your medical well-being is very basic: Don't be a lone wolf! The forlorn creature in the above photograph is a thylacine, sometimes called a Tasmanian wolf. Why did I choose this animal instead of a majestic red or gray wolf? I chose it because the Tasmanian wolf is extinct; if you try to go it alone in a long-term disaster situation, you will be extinct, too. The support of a survival group, even if it's just your extended family, is essential if you are to have any hope of keeping it together when things fall apart.

There will be activities that you would find hard to imagine in an austere setting. You will have to stand watch over your property. You will have to lug gallons of water from the nearest water source. Fill up a 5-gallon bucket with water and walk 100 yards with it (after staying up from midnight to 4:00 a.m. standing outside your house), and you'll get the feel of what you might have to go through on a daily basis.

Being the sole bearer of this burden will negatively affect your health and decrease your chances of long-term survival. Exhausted and sleep-deprived, you will find yourself an easy target not only for marauding gangs but for marauding bacteria as well. Your immune system weakens when exposed to long-term stress, so you will be at risk for illnesses that a well-rested individual could easily weather. Division of labor and responsibility will make a difficult situation more manageable.

You can imagine how much more possible this will be if you have a group of like-minded individuals helping each other. You can't possibly have all the skills needed to do well by yourself, even if you're Daniel Boone. A rugged individualist might be able to eke out a miserable existence in the wilderness alone, but a society can only be rebuilt by a community.

There's no time like the present to communicate, network, and put together a group of like-minded people. The right number of able individuals to assemble for a mutual-assistance group will depend on your retreat and your resources. The ideal group will have people with diverse skills but similar philosophies.

Unless you are already in such a community, you may feel that it is impossible to find and put together a group of people that could help you in times of trouble. Luckily, that isn't the case. You'll find many compatriots in online forums that pertain to preparedness.

It's not enough to just be in a group, however. The people in that group must have regular meetings, decide on priorities, and set things in motion. Put together plan A, plan B, and plan C and work together to make their implementation successful. Keep lines of communication open so that all your group members are kept informed.

Optimize your own health before any catastrophe occurs. If you, as medical caregiver, do not set the example of good health and fitness, how can you expect anyone else to? It's time to practice what you preach. You can accomplish this goal by

- Maintaining a normal weight for your height and age.
- Eating a healthy diet.
- Maintaining good hygiene.
- Keeping physically fit.
- Eliminating unhealthy habits (smoking, and more).
- Managing current medical issues in a timely fashion.

It's important to "tune up" any chronic problems that you might currently have. You'll want to have your blood pressure under control, for example. If you have a bum knee, you might consider getting it repaired surgically so that you can function at maximum efficiency if times get tough. Use modern technology while it is available.

Dental problems should also be managed before bad times make modern dentistry unavailable. Remember how your last toothache affected your work efficiency? If you don't work to achieve all of the above goals, your preparations will be useless.

This plan is important for your mental health as well. Just doing crossword puzzles or reading a newspaper will help keep your mind sharp. Remember that a mind is a terrible thing to waste. Don't waste yours.

If you have bad habits, work to eliminate them. If you damage your heart and lungs by smoking, how will you be able to function in a situation where your fitness and stamina will be continually tested? If you drink alcohol in excess or use drugs, how can you expect anyone to trust your judgment in critical situations?

Paying careful attention to hygiene is also an important factor for your success in times of trouble. Those who fail to maintain sanitary conditions in their retreat will have a difficult time staying healthy. In a collapse, infections usually seen only in underdeveloped countries will become commonplace, and essential medical supplies will include things like soap and bleach.

These two basic strategies, fostering community and practicing preventive medicine and fitness, will take you a long way in your journey to preparedness. They don't cost anything to speak of and will give you the best chance of succeeding if everything else fails.

II.

✚ ✚ ✚

BECOMING A MEDICAL RESOURCE

THE STATUS ASSESSMENT

The first thing that the survival medic should perform in preparation for a collapse situation is a status assessment. The questions below must be asked and answered.

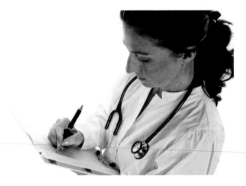

What Will Your Responsibilities Be?

It goes without saying that, as medic, you will be responsible for the medical well-being of your survival community. But what does that mean? It means that, as well as being the chief medical officer, you will take on the following roles:

Chief sanitation officer

It will be your duty to make sure that sanitary conditions at your camp or retreat don't cause the spread of disease among the members. This will be a major issue in an austere setting.

Some of your responsibilities will relate to latrine placement and construction; others will relate to the supervision of appropriate filtering and sterilization of water. Ensurance of proper cleaning of food preparation surfaces will also be very important, as will be the maintenance of good personal and group hygiene.

Chief dental officer

Medical personnel in wartime or in remote locations report that patients arriving at sick call complained of dental problems as much as medical problems. Anyone who has had a bad toothache knows that it affects concentration and, certainly, work efficiency. You will need to know how to deal with dental issues (toothaches, broken teeth, lost fillings) if you are going to be an effective medic.

Chief counselor

It goes without saying that any societal collapse would wreak havoc with people's mindsets. You will have to know how to deal with depression and anxiety as well as cuts and broken bones. You will have to sharpen your communication skills as much as your medical skills.

Medical quartermaster

You've accumulated medical and dental supplies, but when do you break them out and use them? When will you dispense your limited supply of antibiotics? In a survival setting, these items may no longer be manufactured. Careful monitoring of supply stock and usage will give you an idea of your readiness to handle medical emergencies for the long term.

Medical archivist

You are in charge of archiving the medical histories of the people in your group. This record will be useful in remembering all the medical conditions that your people have, their allergies, and medications that they might be taking. If your community is large, it would be almost impossible to memorize all of this information.

Also, your histories of the treatments you have performed on each patient are important to put into writing. One day, you might not be there to render care; your archives will be a valuable resource to the person who is in charge when you're not available.

Medical education resource

You can't be in two places at once, and you will have to make sure that those in your group have some basic medical education. It's important that they can care for injuries or illness while you're away.

These responsibilities are many but may be modified somewhat by the makeup of your group. If you have a pastor or other clergy in your group, they can take some of the burden of counseling away from you. Take whatever help you can get.

How Many People Will You Be Responsible For?

Your store of medical supplies should correlate well with the number of people you will be responsible for. If you have stockpiled five treatment courses of antibiotics, it might be enough for a couple or a sole individual, but it will go fast if you are taking care of twenty people.

Remember that most of those people will be out performing tasks that they aren't used to doing. They will be making campfires, chopping wood and toting gallons of water. You'll see more injuries like sprains and strains, fractures, lacerations, and burns among those people as they perform activities of daily survival.

It only makes sense to accumulate as many supplies as you possibly can. You might wind up dealing with more survivors than you expected; in reality, you almost certainly will. The biggest mistake that the survival medic is likely to make is the underestimation of the number of people who will appear on their doorstep in times of trouble.

Don't be concerned that you have too much stored away. Any "excess" items will always be highly sought after for barter purposes. Food and medical items will be more valuable than silver and gold in hard times. Don't become complacent just because you have a closet full of bandages; they will be used more quickly than you think. Always have more medical items on hand than you think are sufficient for the number of people in your group.

What Special Needs Will You Have to Care For?

The special issues you will deal with depend on who is in your group. The medical needs of children or the elderly are different from an average adult. Women have different health problems than men. You will have to know if group members have a chronic condition, such as asthma or diabetes. Failure to take things like this into account could be catastrophic. For example, would you be prepared if you found out a group member required adult diapers *after* a calamity occurs?

These variables will modify the supplies and medical knowledge you must obtain. Encourage those with special needs to stockpile materials they'll routinely need. Encourage them to have a frank discussion with their physician and obtain extra drug prescriptions in case of emergency (filled in advance).

What Physical Environment Will You Live In?

Is your retreat in a cold climate? If so, you will need to know how to keep people warm and how to treat hypothermia. If you're located in a hot climate, you will need to know how to treat heat stroke. Is your environment wet and humid? People who are chronically wet don't stay healthy, so you will have to have 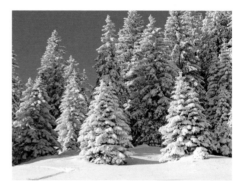 a strategy to keep your group members dry. Are you in a dry, desertlike environment? If you are, you will have to have strategies for providing lots of clean water.

Some people live in areas where all of the above conditions exist at one point or another during the year. These considerations might even factor into where you choose to live if a collapse is imminent.

How Long Do You Expect to Be the Sole Medical Resource?

Some catastrophes, such as major damage from tornadoes or hurricanes, may limit access to medical care for a relatively short period of time. Other events could precipitate a long-term collapse.

The longer you will be the healthcare resource for your group, the more supplies you will have to stockpile and the more varied those supplies should be. If the catastrophe means a few weeks without medical care, you probably can get away without, for example, equipment to extract a diseased tooth. If it's a true collapse, however, that equipment will be quite important. Remember to plan for issues that may occur further down the road, such as birth control for a daughter who has not yet reached puberty.

How Do You Get the Information You Will Need to Be an Effective Healthcare Provider?

A good library of medical, dental, survival, and nutritional books will give you the tools to be an effective medic. Even if you were already a doctor—let's say a general practitioner—you would need various references to learn how to perform surgical procedures that you ordinarily would send to the local surgeon.

Although printed matter is more important off the grid, don't ignore online sources of information. Take advantage of websites with quality medical information. By collecting information you believe will be helpful to your specific situation, you will have a unique store of knowledge that fits your particular needs.

Sites like YouTube.com have thousands of medically oriented videos on just about every topic. They range from suturing wounds to setting a fractured bone to extracting a damaged tooth. To us, seeing things done in real time is always better than just looking at pictures.

How Do You Obtain Medical Training?

There are various ways to get practical training. Almost every municipality gives you access to various courses that would help you function as an effective healthcare provider.

These programs are based around delivering the patient to a hospital as an end result. As medical facilities may not be accessible in the aftermath of a disaster, these classes may not be perfect for a long-term survival situation; nevertheless, you will still learn a lot of useful information.

Although EMT courses are excellent, most of us will not have the time and resources to commit to such intensive training. For most of us, a Red Cross first responder or community emergency response team (CERT) course is the ticket. These programs cover a lot of the same subjects and would certainly represent a good start. The usual course length is 40–80 hours.

Of course, the Red Cross and others provide standard cardio-pulmonary resuscitation (CPR) courses, which everyone should take, whether or not they will have medical responsibility in times of trouble.

Use your spare time to volunteer at the local emergency room. You'll desensitize yourself to seeing blood and injuries and will pick up useful knowledge just by observing.

LIKELY MEDICAL ISSUES YOU WILL FACE

It is important to tailor your education and training to the probable medical issues you will have to treat. By looking at the experience of caregivers in remote settings, you can determine what medical supplies will be needed and prepare yourself for the most likely medical issues.

It wouldn't be unusual to see the following:

- ☤ Trauma
  - Minor musculoskeletal injuries (sprains and strains)
  - Minor trauma (cuts, scrapes)
  - Major traumatic injury (fractures, occasional knife or gunshot wounds)
  - Burn injuries (all degrees)

- ☤ Infections
  - Respiratory infections (pneumonia, bronchitis, influenza, common colds)
  - Diarrheal disease (sometimes in epidemic proportions)
  - Infected wounds
  - Minor infections (urinary infections, "pinkeye")
  - Sexually transmitted diseases
  - Lice, ticks, mosquitoes, and the diseases they carry

- ☤ Allergic reactions
  - Minor (for example, bites or stings from insects)
  - Major (anaphylactic shock)

- ☤ Dental
  - Toothaches
  - Broken or knocked-out teeth
  - Loss of fillings
  - Loose crowns or other dental work

- ☤ Women's issues
  - Pregnancy
  - Miscarriage
  - Birth control

Pregnancy is relatively safe these days, but there was a time in the not too distant past where the announcement of a pregnancy was met as much with concern as joy. Complications—such as miscarriage, bleeding, and infection—took their toll on women, and you must seriously plan to prevent pregnancies, at least until things stabilize.

MEDICAL SKILLS YOU WILL WANT TO LEARN

A very reasonable question for an aspiring medic to ask is "What will I need to know?" The answer is "As much as you're willing to learn!" Using the previous list of likely medical issues will give you a good idea of what skills you'll need. You can expect to deal with lots of ankle sprains, colds, cuts, rashes, and other common medical issues that affect you today. However, you should know how to deal with more significant problems, such as a leg fracture or other traumatic injury. You'll also need to know what medical supplies will be required and how to use them. The effective medic will have learned the following:

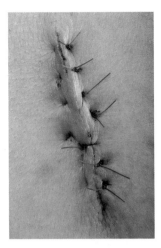

- How to take vital signs, such as pulses, respiration rates and blood pressures.
- How to place wraps and bandages on injuries.
- How to clean and monitor an open wound.
- How to treat varying degrees of burns.
- The indications for use of various drugs and herbal remedies as well as the dosages, frequency of administration, and side effects of those substances. You can't do this on your own; you'll need resources such as the *Physicians' Desk Reference*. This is a weighty volume that comes out yearly and has all the information you'll need to use for both prescription and nonprescription drugs.
- How to perform a normal delivery of a baby and placenta.
- How to splint, pad, and wrap a sprain, dislocation, or fracture.
- How to identify bacterial infectious diseases (such as strep throat).
- How to identify viral infectious diseases (such as influenza).
- How to identify parasitic and protozoal infectious diseases (such as giardiasis).

- How to identify and treat head, pubic, and body lice, as well as insect bites and stings.
- How to identify venomous snakes and treat the effects of their bites, as well as the bites from other animals.
- How to identify and treat various causes of abdominal, pelvic, and chest pain.
- How to treat allergic reactions and anaphylactic shock.
- How to identify and treat sexually transmitted diseases.
- How to evaluate and treat dental disease (such as replace fillings, treat abscesses and perform extractions).
- How to identify and treat skin disease and rashes.
- How to care for the bedridden patient (such as treating bedsores, transport considerations).
- Basic hygiene, nutrition, and sanitary practices. (This couldn't be more important.)
- How to counsel the depressed or anxious patient (common in times of trouble).
- How to insert an intravenous line (IV) line. (EMT classes teach this.)
- How to close a wound.

Actually, more important than knowing how to close a wound is *when* to do so. Most wounds incurred in the outdoors will be dirty wounds, and closing such an injury can lead to bacteria being locked into the tissues, causing infection.

Perhaps the most important skill to obtain is how to prevent injuries and illnesses. Observe simple things, such as whether your people are appropriately dressed for the weather. Make certain to enforce the use of hand and eye protection during work sessions. Learn to recognize situations that place those you are medically responsible for at risk, and you will avoid many injuries and illnesses.

Don't feel that learning all this information is impossible, or that you can't be of benefit if you only learn some of the above. The important thing to do is to learn at least enough to treat some of the more common medical issues.

MEDICAL SUPPLIES

Properly caring for the medical needs of others requires having the right equipment. Imagine a carpenter having to use a steak knife as a saw, or a hunter using a pea shooter instead of a rifle. The same goes for the medic.

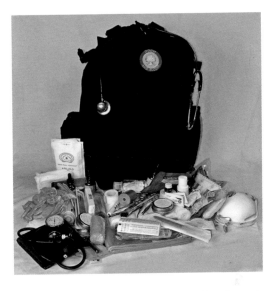

It's important to note that the value of many medical supplies depends largely on the knowledge and skill that the user has obtained through study and practice. A blood pressure cuff isn't very useful to someone who doesn't know how to take a blood pressure. Concentrate on first obtaining items that you can use effectively, and then purchase more advanced equipment as your skills advance.

Don't forget that many items can be improvised; a bandanna may serve as a sling, an ironing board as a stretcher, or thin fishing line and a sewing needle might be useful in sewing up a wound. A careful inspection of your own home would probably turn up things that can be adapted to medical use. Look with a creative eye, and you'll be surprised at the medical issues you are already equipped to deal with.

Sterile vs. Clean

A significant factor in the quality of medical care given in a survival situation is the level of cleanliness of the equipment used.

From a medical standpoint, "sterility" means the complete absence of microbes. Sterile technique involves hand washing with special solutions and the use of sterile instruments, towels, and dressings. When used on a patient, the area immediately around these items is referred to as a "sterile field." The sterile field is closely guarded to prevent contact with anything that could enable microorganisms to invade it.

To guarantee the elimination of all organisms, an autoclave—a type of pressure cooker—is used for instruments, towels, and other items that could come in contact with the patient. All hospitals, clinics, and medical offices clean their equipment with this device. Having a pressure cooker as part of your supplies will enable your instruments to approach the level of sterility required for minor surgical procedures.

Of course, it may be very difficult to achieve a sterile field if you are in an austere environment. In this case, we may only be able to keep things "clean." Techniques for achieving this concentrate on reducing the number of microorganisms that could be transferred from one person to another by medical instruments. Thorough hand washing with soap and hot water is the cornerstone of a clean field.

To maintain a clean area, certain disinfectants are used. Disinfectants are chemical substances that are applied to nonliving objects to destroy microbes. This would include surfaces where you would treat patients or prepare food. Disinfection does not necessarily kill all bugs and, as such, is not as effective as sterilization. An example of a disinfectant would be bleach.

Disinfection removes bacteria, viruses, and other bugs and is sometimes considered the same as decontamination. Decontamination, however, may also include the removal of noxious toxins and could pertain to the elimination of chemicals or radiation. The removal of nonliving toxins, such as radiation, from a surface would, therefore, be decontamination but not disinfection.

It's useful to know the difference between a disinfectant, an antibiotic, and an antiseptic. While disinfectants kill bacteria and viruses on the surface of nonliving tissue, antiseptics kill microbes on living tissue surfaces. Examples of antiseptics include Betadine™, chlorhexidine (Hibiclens), iodine, and benzalkonium chloride (BZK).

Antibiotics are able to destroy microorganisms that live inside the human body. These include drugs such as amoxicillin, doxycycline, metronidazole, and many others. We'll discuss these in detail later in the book.

Medical Kits

Most commercial first-aid kits are fine for the family picnic or a day at the beach, but we discuss serious medical stockpiles here. There are three levels of medical kits that we identify below. The first is a personal-carry or individual first-aid kit, sometimes called an IFAK. Every member of a group can carry this lightweight kit. It enables treatment of some common medical problems encountered in the wilderness or during travel.

The second kit listed below is the family kit, which is mobile, with the items fitting in a standard large backpack. It will suffice as a medical "bug-out" (travel) bag for a couple and their children. It is, in our opinion, the minimum amount of equipment that a head of household would need to handle common emergencies in a long-term survival situation.

The third kit is the community clinic, or everything that a skillful medic will have stockpiled for long-term care of his or her survival family or group.

Don't feel intimidated by the sheer volume of supplies in the clinic version; it would be enough to serve as a reasonably well-equipped field hospital. Few of us have the resources or skills to purchase and effectively use every single item. If you can put together a good family kit, you will have accomplished quite a bit.

The list of items could go on and on, but the important thing is to accumulate supplies and equipment that you will feel competent using in the event of an illness or an injury. Some supplies, such as stretchers and tourniquets, can be improvised using common household items.

It should be noted that many of the advanced items are probably useful only in the hands of an experienced surgeon and could be very dangerous otherwise. In addition, some of the supplies would be more successful in their purpose with an intact power grid. These items represent a wish list of what I would want if I were taking care of an entire community.

You should not feel that the more advanced supply lists are your responsibility to accumulate alone. Your entire group should contribute to stockpiling medical stores, under the medic's coordination. The same goes for all the medical skills that I've listed. To learn everything would be a lifetime of study; more than even most formally trained physicians can accomplish. Concentrate on the items that you are most likely to use regularly.

IFAK or Personal Carry Kit

1 cold pack or hot pack
1 ACE™ wrap (4 inches)
1 Israeli bandage or other compression bandage (6 inches)
1 Celox™ hemostatic agent (stops bleeding)
1 tourniquet
2 eye pads
1 pack (2 sheets) Steri-Strips™
1 nail scissors
1 straight hemostat clamp (5 inches)
1 nylon suture (size 2–0)
1 Super Glue™ or medical glue packet
1 tweezers
1 LED penlight
1 stainless steel bandage scissors (7.25 inches)
20 adhesive bandages (1 inch by 3 inches)
10 adhesive bandages (2 inches by 3 inches)
2 sterile dressings (5 inches by 9 inches)
5 pairs large nitrile gloves
20 nonsterile gauze pads (4 inches by 4 inches)
10 sterile gauze pads (4 inches by 4 inches)
5 nonstick sterile dressings (3 inches by 4 inches)
1 rollgauze sterile dressing
1 Mylar™ solar blanket
1 cloth medical tape (1inch by 10 yards)
1 duct tape (2 inches by 5 yards)
1 triangular bandage with safety pins
1 tube of triple antibiotic ointment
10 alcohol wipes
10 povidone-iodine (Betadine) wipes
6 BZK antimicrobial wipes
2 packets burn gel
6 sting relief towelettes
1 hand sanitizer

Note: Quantities will depend on the number of people for which you are medically responsible.

Family Kit

First-aid reference book
Antibacterial soap and hand sanitizers
Antiseptic and alcohol wipes
Gauze dressing (various sizes—sterile and nonsterile)
Gauze rolls (Kerlix, etc.)
Nonstick pads (Telfa)
Triangular bandages or bandannas
Safety pins (large)
Moldable splints
Israeli battle dressings or other compression bandage
Adhesive Band-Aids™ (various sizes and shapes)
Large absorbent pads (ABD, etc.)
Neck collar
Medical tape (Elastoplast, silk, paper varieties; 1 inch and 2 inches)
Duct tape
Tourniquet
Moleskin or Spenco 2nd Skin™ blister kit
Cold packs, heat packs, hot water bottle (reusable if possible)
Cotton eye pads, patches
Eye wash, eye pads
Cotton swabs (Q-tips™), cotton balls
Disposable nitrile gloves (hypoallergenic)
Face masks (surgical and n95)
Tongue depressors
Bandage scissors (all-metal are best)
Tweezers
Magnifying glass
Headlamp or penlight
Stethoscope
Blood pressure cuff
Irrigation syringe (60–100 cc)
Kelly clamp (straight and curved)
Needle holder
Nylon or silk sutures (sizes 2–0, 4–0) and/or stapler kit
Scalpel or field knife

Chest seals
Styptic pencil
Hemostatic agents (Celox or QuikClot™ powder)
Saline solution (liter bottle or smaller)
Steri-Strips or butterfly closures, thin and thick sizes
Tincture of benzoin (glue to hold Steri-Strips in place long-term)
Survival sheet/solar blanket
Biohazard bags
Thermometer
Antiseptic solutions (Betadine, Hibiclens, etc.)
Hydrogen peroxide (3 percent)
Benzalkonium chloride wipes
Witch hazel
Antibiotic ointment
Antacids
Sunblock
Lip balms
Insect repellant
Ammonia inhalants
Hydrocortisone cream (1 percent)
Lidocaine cream (2.5 percent; local anesthetic)
Acetaminophen/ibuprofen/aspirin
Diphenhydramine (Benadryl™) or loratadine (Claritin™)
Loperamide (Imodium™)
Pseudoephedrine (Sudafed™)
Bismuth Subsalicylate (Pepto-Bismol™)
RID™ Lice Killing Shampoo, Fels-Naptha, or Zanfel soap
Soap for general use
Oral rehydration packs (or make them from scratch)
Water purification filter or tablets
Gold Bond foot powder
Silvadene™ cream (for burns)
Oral antibiotics
Epinephrine (EpiPen™, a prescription injection for severe allergic reactions)
Zofran (for nausea and vomiting-prescription)

Birth control accessories (condoms, birth control pills, etc.)
Herbal teas, tinctures, salves, and essential oils
Raw, unprocessed honey

Dental Tray:
    Cotton pellets and rolls
    Dental mirror
    Dental scraper, toothpicks
    Dental floss
    Dental wax
    Clove bud oil
    Zinc oxide
    Commercial dental kits (Dentemp, Cavit™)
    Hanks' solution
    Chromic suture (size 4–0)
    Needle holder
    ActCel™ oral hemostatic agent (stops dental bleeding)
    Extraction equipment (forceps and elevators)
    Gloves, masks, and eye protection

Community Clinic Supply List

For a long-term care center

Obtain all of the above in larger quantities, plus the following:

Extensive medical library
Treatment table
Plaster of Paris cast kits (4–6 inches)
Naso-oropharyngeal airway tubes
Nasal airways
Resuscitation facemask with one-way valve
Resuscitation bag (Ambu™ bag)
Endotracheal tube/laryngoscope (enables you to breathe for patient)
Portable defibrillator
Blood pressure cuff
Stethoscopes
CPR shield
Otoscope and ophthalmoscope
Urine test strips
Pregnancy test kits
Sterile drapes
Air splints
SAM splints
Scrub suits, goggles, or face shields
Foldable stretchers
Paracord (various uses)
Triage tags (for mass casualty incidents)
IV equipment:

- Normal saline solution bags
- Dextrose and normal saline (50 percent) IV solution bags
- IV tubing sets
- Syringes (2, 5, 10, and 20 ml)
- Needles (gauges 20–24)
- IV kits (gauges 16–24)

- Paper tape (½ inch and 1 inch)
- IV stands
- Saline solution for irrigation (can be made at home as well)

Penrose drains (to allow blood and pus to drain from wounds)
Foley urinary catheters (sizes 18, 20)
Urine bags and enema bags
Nasogastric tubes (to pump a stomach)
Pressure cooker (to sterilize instruments, etc.)

Prescription Medications

Medrol dose packs
Antibiotic and anesthetic eye and ear drops
Oral contraceptive pills
Metronidazole
Amoxicillin
Cephalexin
Ciprofloxacin
Doxycycline
Clindamycin
Sulfamethoxazole/trimethoprin
Ceftriaxone
Diazepam
Alprazolam
Oxytocin
Percocet™
Morphine sulfate or Demerol™

NATURAL REMEDIES

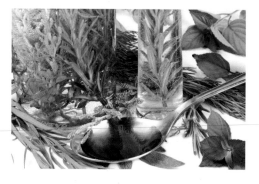

There are many issues that are best handled with the support of the latest technology and modern equipment and facilities. Sure enough, I've just spent the last chapter telling you to stock up on all sorts of high-tech items (even defibrillators!) and, indeed, many of these things are indispensable when it comes to dealing with certain medical conditions.

Unfortunately, you probably will not have the resources needed to stockpile a massive medical arsenal. Even if you are able to do so, your supplies will last only a certain amount of time. You may be shocked at the rapidity with which precious medications and other items are used up.

One solution is to grossly overstock on commonly used medical supplies, but even large stockpiles will eventually dry up when dealing with the common issues you'll encounter. Therefore, you will need a way to produce substances that will have a medical benefit. The plants in your own backyard or nearby woods would be the best place to start.

Physicians have occupied different niches in society over the ages, from priests during the time of the pharaohs, to slaves and barbers in imperial Rome and the Dark Ages, and artists during the Renaissance. All of these ancient healers used different methods, but they had one thing in common: They understood the importance of natural products for medicinal purposes. If they needed more of a particular plant than occurred in their native environment, they cultivated it. They learned to make teas, tinctures, and salves containing these products and how best to use them to treat illness. If modern medical care is no longer available one day, we will have to take advantage of their experience.

An example is salicin, a natural pain reliever found in the under bark of willows, poplar, and aspen trees. In the nineteenth century, we first developed a process to commercially produce aspirin (salicylic acid) from these trees.

Natural remedies should be integrated into the medical toolbox of anyone willing to take responsibility for the well-being of others. Why not use all the tools that are available to you? At one point or another, the medicinal herbs and plants you grow in your garden may be all you have.

Natural substances can be used in "home remedies" through several methods, including the following:

Teas: a hot drink made by infusing the dried, crushed leaves of a plant in boiling water.

Tinctures: plant extracts made by soaking herbs in a liquid (such as water, grain alcohol, or vinegar) for a specified length of time, then straining and discarding the plant material (also known as a "decoction").

Essential oils: liquids comprised of highly concentrated aromatic mixtures of natural compounds obtained from plants. These are typically made by a process called "distillation"; most have long shelf lives.

Salves: highly viscous or semisolid substances used on the skin (also known as an ointment, unguent, or balm).

Some of these products may also be ingested directly or diluted in solutions. A major benefit of home remedies is that they usually have fewer side effects than commercially produced drugs. It is the obligation of the group medic to obtain a working knowledge of how to use and, yes, grow these plants. For more detailed information on individual herbs, see the latest edition of our comprehensive book *The Survival Medicine Handbook*.

Another alternative therapy thought by some to boost immune systems and treat illness is colloidal silver. Colloidal silver products are made of tiny silver particles, silver ions, or silver combined with protein, all suspended in a liquid. Silver compounds were used to treat infections before the development of antibiotics.

Colloidal silver products are usually marketed as dietary supplements that are taken by mouth. They also come in forms that can be applied to the skin, where they are thought to improve healing by preventing infection. It should be noted that long-term ingestion of silver may result in a condition known as argyria. This rare condition is mostly a cosmetic, causing skin to turn blue.

Ionic silver (Ag+) and silver particles in concentration have been shown to have an antimicrobial effect in certain laboratory studies. Physicians use wound dressings containing silver sulfadiazine (Silvadene) to help prevent infection. Wound dressings containing silver are being used more and more often because of the increase in bacterial resistance to antibiotics.

You should know that the US Food and Drug Administration (FDA) has banned colloidal silver sellers from claiming any therapeutic or preventive value. As a result, it cannot be marketed as preventing or treating any illness. More evidence is warranted before silver becomes a standard part of the medical arsenal.

THE PHYSICAL EXAM

By reading this book, you have made the decision to take responsibility for the medical well-being of your family in the aftermath of a disaster. Therefore, it will be necessary to build a store of knowledge of how to evaluate a patient and make a diagnosis.

You will have to put your (gloved) hands on them and be able to look for physical signs of illness or evaluate wounds in a systematic manner. Sometimes the problem is obvious in seconds; other times, you will have to examine the entire body to determine the problem. During an exam, always communicate to your patient who you are, what you are doing, and why. Remain calm and be very careful about forcing them to move or perform an action that is beyond their capability.

The most basic information is obtained by checking the vital signs. This includes the following:

Pulse rate. This can be taken by using two fingers to press on the side of the neck or the inside of the wrist (by the base of the thumb). A normal pulse rate at rest is 60–100 beats per minute. You may choose to feel the pulse for, say, 15 seconds and multiply the number you get by 4 to get beats per minute. A full minute would be more accurate, however. You will find that most people who are agitated from having suffered an injury will have a high pulse rate (tachycardia).

Respiration rate. This is best evaluated for 1 full minute to get an accurate reading. The normal adult rate at rest is 12–18 breaths per minute, somewhat more for children. Note any unusual aspects, such as wheezing or gurgling noises. A respiration rate of more than 20 breaths per minute is a sign of a person in distress and is known as tachypnea.

Blood pressure. Blood pressure is a measure of the work the heart has to do to pump blood throughout the body. You're looking for a pressure of less than 140/90 at rest. Blood pressure may be high after extreme physical exertion but goes back down after a short while. Of course, some people have high blood pressure as a chronic condition. A very low blood pressure may be seen in a person who has hemorrhaged or is in shock. Instructions on how to take a blood pressure can be found in the high blood pressure section of the book.

Mental status. You want to know that your patient is alert and, therefore, can respond to questions and commands. Ask your patient what happened. If they seem disoriented, ask simple questions like their name, where they are, or what year it is. Note whether the patient appears lethargic or agitated. Some patients may appear unconscious but respond to a spoken command, for example, "Hey! Open your eyes!" If no response, see if the patient reacts to a stimulus, such as gentle pressure on their breastbone. If they don't, something very serious is going on.

Body temperature. Take the patient's temperature to verify that they don't have a fever. A normal temperature will range from 97.5 to 99.0 degrees. (*Note:* All degrees of temperature in this book are expressed in Fahrenheit. To convert to Celsius, use the following formula: multiply by 1.8 and add 32.) A significant fever is defined as a temperature above 100.4 degrees). Very low temperatures (less than 95 degrees may indicate cold-related illness, also known as hypothermia. On the opposite hand is heat stroke (hyperthermia), where the temperature may rise above 105 degrees.

Once you've taken the vital signs and determined that there is no obvious injury, perform a general exam from head to toe in an organized fashion. Touch the patient's skin. Is it hot or cold, moist or dry? Is there redness, or is the patient pale? Examine the head area and work your way down. Are there any bumps on the head; are they bleeding from the nose, mouth, or ears? Evaluate the eyes and see if they are reddened. Use a light source to see if the pupils respond equally to light.

Have the patient open their mouth and check for redness, sores, or dental issues with a light source and a tongue depressor. Check the neck for evidence of injury, and feel the back of the head and neck, especially the neck bones (vertebrae).

Take your stethoscope and listen to the chest, which is called "auscultation." Do you hear the patient breathing as you place the instrument over different areas of each lung? Are there noises that shouldn't be there? Practice listening on healthy people to get a good idea of what clear lungs should sound like. Abnormal sounds would include wheezing, gurgles, and crackles.

Listen to the heart and see if the heartbeat is regular or irregular in rhythm. Check along the ribs for rough areas that might signify a fracture. Check the armpits (also known as the axilla) for masses. Perform a breast exam by moving your fingers in a circular motion over the breast tissue, starting from the periphery near the axilla and ending at the nipple.

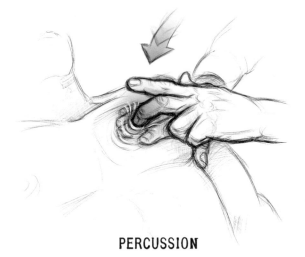

PERCUSSION

Palpate the abdomen, which means press on the abdomen with your open hand. Is there pain? Is the belly soft, or is it rigid and swollen? Do you feel any masses? Use your stethoscope to listen to the gurgling of bowel sounds. Lack of bowel sounds may indicate lack of intestinal motility; excessive bowel sounds may be seen in some diarrheal disease. Place your open hand on the different quadrants of the abdomen and tap on your middle finger. This is called "percussion." The abdomen will sound hollow normally, but dull where there might be a mass. Press down on the right side below the rib cage to determine if the liver is enlarged (you won't feel it if it isn't). An enlarged spleen will appear as a mass on the left side under the bottom of the rib cage.

Check along the patient's spine for evidence of pain or injury. Pound lightly with a closed hand on each side of the back below the last rib, where the kidneys are; injury or infection would cause this action to be very painful to the patient.

Check each extremity by feeling the muscle groups for pain or decreased range of motion. Make sure the patient's circulation is good by checking the color on the tips of the fingers and toes. Poor circulation will make these areas white or blue in color. Check for sensation by lightly tapping with a safety pin. Place your hands on the patient's thighs and ask them to lift up, to check for normal strength and tone. Ask them to grasp your fingers with each hand; then, try to pull your hand away. If you can't, that's good.

If you draw a line vertically down the length of the human body, each side is essentially the same (with a few internal exceptions). This means that, if you are uncertain whether a limb is injured or deformed, you can compare it with the other side. The strength on each side should be about equal.

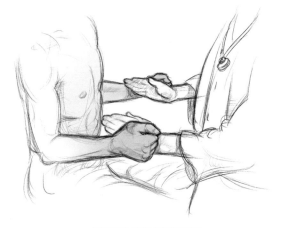

STRENGTH TESTING

These are just some basics. Certainly, there's a lot more to a physical exam than we just described, but practicing exams on others will give you experience. As time goes by, you'll get the feel of what is normal and what isn't.

THE MASS CASUALTY INCIDENT

You've just read about performing a physical exam. Most of these exams will be unhurried and routine, but, occasionally, you will have to make some quick decisions. For major trauma, it is important to take note of the "golden hour"—

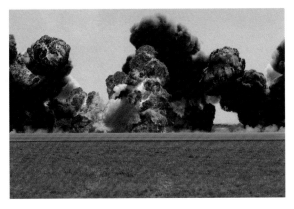

the first hour after the victim's injury, when his or her chance of survival is highest. A victim's chance of survival decreases significantly if not treated within that hour. It then worsens with every thirty minutes that pass without care.

Usually, the healthcare provider will be dealing with one ill or injured individual at a time. There may be a day, however, when you find yourself confronted with an emergency scenario in which multiple people are injured. This is referred to as a mass casualty incident (MCI).

A masscasualty incident is any event in which your medical resources are inadequate for the number and severity of injuries incurred. MCIs can be quite variable in their presentation and can include any of the following:

- Doomsday scenario events, such as nuclear weapon detonations
- Terrorist acts, such as occurred on 9/11 or in Oklahoma City
- Consequences of a storm, such as a tornado or hurricane
- Consequences of civil unrest
- A mass transit mishap (train derailment, plane crash, etc.)
- A car accident with, for example, three people significantly injured and only one ambulance

The effective medical management of any of the events listed above requires rapid and accurate triage. Triage, which comes from the French word *trier* ("to sort"), is the process by which medical personnel can rapidly assess and prioritize a number of injured individuals, thereby doing the most good for the most people. Note that I didn't say, "Give the best possible care to *each* individual victim."

Evaluating an MCI Scene

Your initial actions at the scene of an MCI may determine the outcome of the emergency response. The following constitute the five S's of evaluating an MCI scene:

- Safety
- Sizing up
- Sending for help
- Setup of areas
- Simple triage and rapid treatment (START), a term used in triage

1. Safety assessment. In the Middle East, an insidious strategy on the part of terrorists is the use of primary and secondary bombs. The main bomb causes the most casualties, and the second bomb is timed to go off or is triggered just as the medical and security personnel arrive.

Many medical professionals wince when I talk about not approaching the injured in a hostile setting. Remember that your primary goal as medic is your own self-preservation; keeping the medical personnel alive is likely to save more lives down the road.

As you arrive on the scene, be as certain as possible that there is no ongoing threat. Do not rush in there until it is clear that you and your helpers are safe.

2. Sizing up the scene. Ask yourself the following questions:

- What's the situation? Is this a mass-transit crash? Did a building on fire collapse?
- How many injuries and how severe? Are there a few victims or dozens? Are there others who can help?
- Are the victims all together or spread out over a wide area?
- What are possible nearby areas for transport and treatment of the injured?
- Are there areas open enough for vehicles to come through to help transport victims?

3. Sending for help. If modern medical care is available, call 911 and say (for example), "I am calling to report a mass casualty incident involving a multivehicle auto accident at the intersection of Hollywood and Vine. At least seven people are injured and will require medical attention. There may be people trapped in their cars, and one vehicle is on fire."

In three sentences, you have informed the authorities that a mass casualty event has occurred, what type of event it was, where it occurred, an approximate number of patients that may need care, and the types of care or equipment that may be needed.

If you are the only one there, get your phone or other communication device and notify others of the situation and what you'll need in terms of personnel and supplies. If you are not medically trained, contact the person who is the group medic. The most experienced medical person is the incident commander.

4. Setup. Determine likely areas for victims of various levels of illness (see below) to be further evaluated and treated. Also, determine the appropriate entry and exit points for victims that need immediate transport to medical facilities, if they exist.

5. START. The first round of triage, known as "primary triage," should be fast (30 seconds per patient, if possible) and does not involve extensive treatment of injuries. It should be focused on identifying the triage level of each patient. Evaluation in primary triage consists mostly of quick evaluation of respiration (or the lack thereof), perfusion (adequacy of circulation), and mental status. Other than controlling massive bleeding and clearing airways, very little treatment is performed in primary triage.

Although there is no international standard for this, triage levels are usually determined by color:

> **Immediate (red tag)** – The victim needs immediate medical care and will not survive without rapid treatment (for example, a major hemorrhagic wound or internal bleeding). This person has top priority.

> **Delayed (yellow tag)** – The victim needs medical care within 2–4 hours. Injuries may become life threatening if ignored (for example, open fracture of femur without major hemorrhage) but can wait until patients with red tags are treated.

Minimal (green tag) – Generally stable and ambulatory ("walking wounded") but may need some medical care (for example, broken fingers, sprained wrist).

Expectant (black tag) – The victim is either deceased or is not expected to live (for example, open skull fracture with brain damage, or multiple penetrating chest wounds).

Knowing this patient marking system easily enables a caregiver to understand the urgency of a patient's situation. It should go without saying that, in a power-down situation without modern medical care, a lot of red tags and even some yellow tags will become black tags. It will be difficult to save someone with major internal bleeding without surgical intervention.

Let's go through an example of a mass casualty incident and discuss how triage duties should be performed.

Primary Triage: MCI Scenario

Here's our hypothetical scenario: You are walking down the street when you hear an explosion. You are the first one to arrive at the scene, and you are alone. There are about twenty people down, and there is blood everywhere. What do you do?

Referring back to the five S's, let's assume that you have already determined the *safety* of the current situation and *sized-up* the scene. There appears to have been a bomb that exploded. There are no hostiles nearby, as far as you can tell, and there is no evidence of incoming ordnance. Therefore, you believe that you and other responders are not in danger. The injuries are significant, and the victims are all in one area.

The incident occurred on a main thoroughfare, so there are ways in and out. You have *sent* a call for help and described the scene, and have received replies from several group members, including a former intensive care unit (ICU) nurse who is contacting everyone else with medical experience. The area is relatively open, so you can *set up* areas for various triage categories. Now you can *START*.

You will call out as loudly as possible: "I'm here to help, everyone who can get up and walk and needs medical attention, get up and move to the sound of my voice. If you are uninjured and can help, follow me."

You're lucky, thirteen of the twenty, mostly from the periphery of the blast, sit up, or at least try to. Ten can stand, and eight go to the area you designated for walking wounded. These people have cuts and scrapes, and a couple of them are limping; one has obviously broken an arm. Two bruised but sturdy individuals join you. By communicating, you have made your job as temporary incident commander easier by identifying the walking wounded (green tags) and getting some immediate help. You still have ten victims down.

You then go to the closest victim on the ground. Start right where you are and go to the next nearest victim in turn. In this way, you will triage faster and more effectively than trying to figure out who needs help the most from a distance or going in a haphazard pattern.

Let's cheat just a little and say that you happen to have what are known as "SMART" tags in your pack. SMART tags are handy tickets that enable you to mark a particular triage level on a patient. Once you identify a victim's triage level, you remove a portion of the end of the tag until you reach the appropriate color and place it around the patient's wrist.

You could, instead, use colored markers or numbers placed on the victims' foreheads. If you use numbers, follow this coding:

- Priority 1—immediate/red
- Priority 2—delayed/yellow
- Priority 3—minimal/green
- Priority 4—dead or expectant/black

It is important to remember that you are triaging, not treating. The only treatments in START will be stopping massive bleeding, opening airways, and elevating the legs in case of shock. As you go from patient to patient, stay calm, and identify who you are and that you're there to help. Your goal is to find out who will need help most urgently (red tags). You will be assessing respiration, perfusion, and mental status (RPM).

   ⚕ **Respiration:** Is your patient breathing? If not, tilt the head back or insert an oral airway if available. (*Note:* In modern emergency care, the neck is not moved unless a cervical spine injury has been ruled out; in an MCI triage situation, the rule is temporarily suspended.) If you have an open airway and no breathing, that victim is tagged black. If the victim breathes once an airway is restored or is breathing more than 30 times a minute, tag red. If the victim is breathing normally, move to perfusion.

☤ **Perfusion:** Determine how normal the blood flow or circulation is. Check for a (wrist or neck) pulse. Alternatively, press on the nail bed or pad of a finger firmly and quickly remove. It will go from white to normal color in less than 2 seconds if there is good perfusion. This is referred to as the capillary refill time (CRT). If there is no pulse, or it takes longer than 2 seconds for the color to return to pink, tag red. If a pulse is present and CRT is normal, move on to checking mental status.

☤ **Mental status:** Can the patient follow simple commands ("open your eyes," "what's your name?")? If the patient is breathing and has normal perfusion but is unconscious or disoriented, tag red. Tag patients yellow if they can understand you and follow commands but can't get up, green if they can. Remember that, as a consequence of the explosion, some victims may not be able to hear you well.

It might be easier to remember all this by just thinking "30–2–Can Do": 30 (respirations), 2 (CRT), Can Do (Commands).

If there is any doubt as to the category, always tag the highest priority triage level—red. Once you have identified someone as triage level red, tag them and move immediately to the next patient unless you have major bleeding to stop. Any one RPM check that does not meet the 30–2–Can Do rule tags the victim as red. For example, if someone wasn't breathing but began breathing once you repositioned the airway, tag red, and stop further evaluation if the person is not hemorrhaging. Elevate the legs if you suspect shock, then move to the next patient.

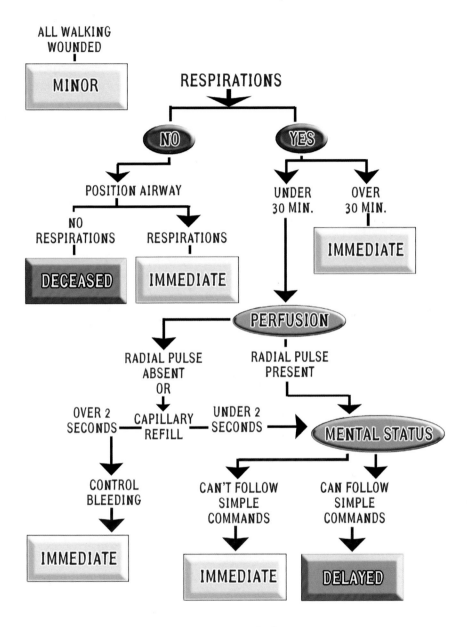

ALL WALKING WOUNDED

MINOR

RESPIRATIONS

NO

YES

POSITION AIRWAY

UNDER 30 MIN.

OVER 30 MIN.

NO RESPIRATIONS

RESPIRATIONS

IMMEDIATE

DECEASED

IMMEDIATE

PERFUSION

RADIAL PULSE ABSENT OR

RADIAL PULSE PRESENT

OVER 2 SECONDS

CAPILLARY REFILL

UNDER 2 SECONDS

MENTAL STATUS

CONTROL BLEEDING

CAN'T FOLLOW SIMPLE COMMANDS

CAN FOLLOW SIMPLE COMMANDS

IMMEDIATE

IMMEDIATE

DELAYED

TRIAGE CASCADE

Now, let's return to our mass casualty event. You have identified eight walking wounded and moved them to a designated area. Your two uninjured helpers are an able-bodied man and woman. The woman knows how to take a pulse. Let's say you have no medical equipment with you other than some oral airways and triage tags to work with. We describe below how to triage your ten victims, starting with the closest.

Victim 1. Male in his thirties, complains of pain in his left leg (obviously fractured), respirations are 24 times per minute, pulse strong, CRT is 1 second, no excessive bleeding.

Respirations are within acceptable range (fewer than 30); pulse and CRT is normal. The patient complains of pain and is communicating where it hurts, so mental status is probably normal. This patient is tagged yellow: needs care but will not die if there is a reasonable (2–4 hour) delay. Move on.

Victim 2. Female in her fifties, bleeding from nose, ears, and mouth. Trying to sit up but can't, respirations are 20, pulse is present, CRT is 1 second, not responding to your commands.

This victim has a significant head injury but is stable from the standpoint of respirations and perfusion. As her mental status is impaired, tag red (immediate). Move on.

Victim 3. Teenage girl bleeding heavily from her right thigh, respirations are 32, pulse is thready, CRT is 2.5 seconds, follows commands.

This victim is seriously hemorrhaging, one of the reasons to treat during triage. Respirations are elevated and perfusion is impaired. You have your unskilled male helper place his hands on the bleeding and apply pressure, preferably using his shirt or bandanna as a dressing. Tag red. As the patient is already tagged red, you don't really have to assess mental status. You and your female helper move on.

Victim 4. Another teenage girl, small laceration on forehead, says she can't move her legs. Respirations are 20, pulse is strong, CRT is 1 second.

Probable spinal injury but otherwise stable and can communicate. Tag yellow. Move on.

Victim 5. Male in his twenties, head wound, respirations absent. Airway repositioned, still no breathing.

If he is not breathing, you will reposition his head and place an airway. This fails to restart his breathing. This patient is deceased for all intents and purposes. Tag black and move on.

Victim 6. Male in his forties, burns on face, chest, and arms. Respirations are 22, pulse is 100, CRT is 1.5 seconds, follows commands.

This victim has significant burns over large areas of his body, but is breathing well and has normal perfusion. Mental status is unimpaired, so you tag yellow and move on.

Victim 7. Teenage boy, multiple cuts and abrasions but not hemorrhaging, says he can't breathe, respirations are 34, radial pulse (the pulse of the radial artery palpated at the wrist) is present, CRT is 2.5 seconds.

This victim doesn't look too bad but is having trouble breathing and has questionable perfusion. Mental status is unimpaired, but he likely has other issues, perhaps internal bleeding. You tag red (due to respirations greater than 30 and impaired perfusion). Move on.

Victim 8. Female in her twenties, burns on neck and face, respirations are 22, pulse is present, CRT is 1 second, asks to get up and can walk, although with a limp.

Obviously injured, this young woman is otherwise stable and communicating. With assistance, she is able to stand up, and can walk by herself. She becomes another of the walking wounded: tag green. Point her to the other green victims and move on.

Victim 9. Elderly woman, bleeding profusely from an amputated right arm (level of forearm), respirations are 36, pulse on other wrist is absent, CRT is 3 seconds, unresponsive.

The victims is obviously in dire straits, so you use your shirt as a tourniquet and have your helper apply pressure on the bleeding area. Tag red and move on.

Victim 10. Male child, multiple penetrating injuries, no respirations. Airway repositioned, starts breathing. Radial pulse is absent, CRT is 2 seconds, unresponsive.

You initially think this child is deceased, but you follow protocol and reposition his airway by tilting his head back. In normal circumstances you would be very reluctant to do this because of the possibility of a neck injury. An MCI is one of the few circumstances where you don't worry about cervical spine injuries in making your assessment. To your surprise, he starts breathing even without an oral airway, so you tag him red. If he is bleeding heavily from his injuries, you apply pressure and wait for the additional help you originally requested to arrive.

You have just performed triage on twenty victims, including the walking wounded, in ten minutes or less. Help begins to arrive, including the ICU nurse that you contacted initially. You are no longer the most experienced medical resource at the scene, and you are relieved of incident command. The nurse begins the process of assigning areas where secondary triage and treatment can occur for victims with yellow, red, and black tags.

There is still much to do, but you have identified those victims who need the most urgent care. In a normal situation, modern medical facilities will already have ambulances and trained personnel with lots of equipment on the scene. In an off-grid setting, however, the prognosis for many of the victims is grave. Go over our list of victims and see who you think would survive if modern medical care is not available. Many of the red tags and even some of the yellow tags would be in serious danger of dying from their wounds.

PATIENT TRANSPORT

Before deciding whether to move a patient, stabilize them as much as possible. This means stopping all bleeding, splinting, orthopedic injuries, and verifying that the person is breathing normally. If you cannot ensure this, consider having a group member get the supplies needed to support the patient before you move them. Have as many helpers available to assist you as you can. The most important thing to remember is that you want to carry out the evacuation with the least trauma to your patient and yourself.

An important medical supply to have in this circumstance is a stretcher. Many good commercially produced stretchers are available, but improvised stretchers can be put together without too much effort. Even an ironing board can become an effective transport device. A person with a spinal injury should be rolled onto a stretcher without bending their neck or back, if at all possible.

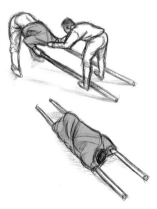

SHIRT STRETCHER

Other options include taking two long sticks or poles and inserting coats or shirts through them to handle the weight of the victim. If the rescuer grasps both poles, a helper could pull their coat off. This automatically moves the coat onto the poles. Lengths of paracord or rope can also be crisscrossed to form an effective stretcher.

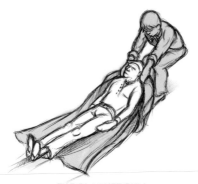

THE BLANKET PULL

If you must pull a person to safety, grasp their coat or shirt at the shoulders with both hands, allowing their head to rest on your forearms. You could also place a blanket under the patient, and grasp the end of the blanket near their head and pull. Again, if you are uncertain about the extent of any spinal injuries, do your best to avoid bending the body or neck during transport.

If your patient can be carried, there are various methods available. The "fireman's carry" is effective and keeps the victim's torso relatively level and stable. If the patient is unconscious, this process is easier if they are carefully positioned so as to lie on their stomach. You can lift by "hugging" the victim under their arms and putting your dominant leg between their bent legs for support. You would then grasp the person's right wrist with your left hand and place it over your right shoulder. Keeping your back straight, place your right hand between their legs and around the right thigh. Using your leg muscles to lift, rising up; you should end up with their torso over your back and their right thigh resting over your right shoulder. Their left arm and leg will hang behind your back if you have done it correctly. Adjust their weight so as to cause the least strain.

Another option is the "pack-strap carry." With your patient behind you, grasp both arms and cross them on the front of your chest. If squatting, keep your back straight and use your legs and back muscles to lift the victim. Bend slightly so that the person's weight is on your hips and lift them off the ground.

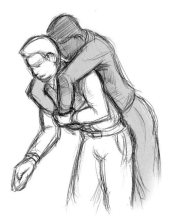

PACK STRAP CARRY

If you have the luxury of an assistant, you might consider placing your patient, if conscious, on a chair and carrying them using their front legs and the back of the chair. This constitutes a sitting "stretcher." Another two-person carry involves one rescuer wrapping their arms around the victim's chest from behind while the second rescuer (facing away from the patient) grabs the patient's legs behind each knee. This is done in a squatting position, using the leg muscles to lift the patient.

It's important to remember this simple acronym when pulling or carrying a person: B.A.C.K, which stands for the following:

Back straight. Muscles and discs can handle more weight safely when the back is straight.

Avoid twisting. Joints can be damaged when twisting.

Close to body. Avoid reaching to pick up a load, as it causes more strain on muscles and joints.

Keep stable. The more rotation and jerking, the more pressure on the discs and muscles.

III.

+ + +

HYGIENE AND SANITATION

HYGIENE-RELATED MEDICAL PROBLEMS

In nature, many animals make specific efforts to preen and groom themselves. Their instinctual tendency to stay clean keeps them healthy. Time and effort spent in remaining clean translates into resistance to disease. When humans are under stress, attention to hygiene suffers because all available energy must be directed to activities of daily survival.

As the medic, you will have some control over the likelihood that your family or group will be exposed to unsanitary conditions. Indeed, your diligence in this matter is one of the major factors that will determine your success as a caregiver. Strict enforcement of good sanitation and hygiene policies will do more to keep your family healthy than anything that any medical doctor can do.

In a situation where there is no access to common cleansing items, such as soap or laundry detergent, the goal of staying clean is difficult to achieve, even with the best of intentions. Therefore, accumulation of these items in quantity is in your best interest.

Cleanliness issues extend to many areas, such as dental care and foot care. The dirtier and wetter we get, the more prone we are to problems such as infections or infestations. With careful attention to hygiene, we can avoid many medical issues, as we discuss in this section.

LICE AND TICKS

Lice

A common health problem pertaining to poor hygiene is louse infestation, also known as "pediculosis." Lice are wingless insects that are found on many species. On humans, there are three types: head, body, and pubic. Lice serve as a 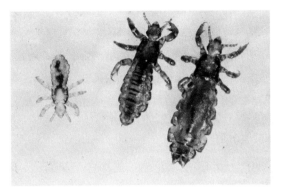 vehicle to transmit some diseases, causing major implications for entire families. Sometimes itching caused by lice leads to breaks in the skin, which enables other infections to develop.

Although it is thought that human lice evolved from organisms on gorillas and chimpanzees, they are, generally speaking, species specific. That means that you cannot get lice from your dog, like you could get fleas. You get them only from other humans.

Lice spread rapidly in crowded, unsanitary conditions or where close personal contact is unavoidable. These conditions occur, for example, in many schools where children come into contact with each other during the course of the day (head lice, mostly). The sharing of personal items can also lead to louse infestations; combs, articles of clothing, pillows, and towels that are used by multiple individuals are common ways that lice are spread.

Adult head lice (*Pediculus humanus capitis*) are greyish-white and can reach the size of a small sesame seed. Infestation with head lice can cause itching and, sometimes, a rash. However, this type of lice is not a carrier of any other disease. Even in developed countries, head lice are relatively common, with 6–12 million cases a year in the United States, mostly among young children.

With their less developed immune systems, kids sometimes don't even know they have them; adults are usually kept scratching and irritated unless treated.

The diagnosis is made by identifying the presence of the louse or its "nits" (eggs). Nits look like small bits of dandruff that are stuck to hairs. A fine-tooth comb run through the hair is a good method to find adult lice and nits. Special combs are used to remove as many lice as possible before treatment and to check for them afterwards. Many prefer the metal nit combs sold at pet stores to plastic ones sold at pharmacies.

You will find that the nits are firmly attached to the hair shaft about one-quarter inch from the scalp. Nits will generally appear as yellow or white and oval-shaped. Nits may be easier to remove by applying olive oil to the comb.

Body lice (*Pediculus humanus corporis*) are latecomers compared with head lice, probably appearing with the advent of humans wearing clothes. As the concept of cleaning clothes occurred quite later, the constant contact with dirty garb caused frequent infestations.

This may be a common issue with the homeless today but will likely be an epidemic in a survival situation when regular bathing and clothes washing becomes problematic. Body lice are slightly larger than head lice; they also differ in that they live on clothes, using the body only to feed. They are sturdier than their cousins and can live without human contact for thirty days or so.

Removal and, preferably, destruction of the infested clothing is the appropriate strategy here. Using medication is sometimes unnecessary, as the lice have left with the clothes (don't bet on it, however). Body lice, unlike head lice, are associated with infectious diseases such as typhus, trench fever, and epidemic relapsing fever. Continuous exposure to body lice may lead to areas on the skin that are hardened and deeply pigmented.

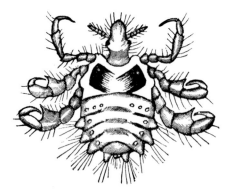

Crab louse

Pubic infestations may be caused by either lice or mites. Pubic lice (*Pthirus pubis*), also known as "crabs," usually start in the pubic region but may eventually extend anywhere there is hair, even the eyelashes. They are most commonly passed by sexual contact. Severe itching is the main symptom and can involve the axillary (armpit) hair or even the eyelashes.

Although they are sometimes seen in a patient as a sexually transmitted disease because they are usually transferred from one person to another through sexual activity, pubic lice do not actually transmit other illnesses. It should be noted that pubic lice constitute one of the few "sexually transmitted diseases"™ that is not prevented by the use of a condom.

Scabies is different from crabs and is caused by tiny eight-legged organisms called mites (*Sarcoptes scabiei*), not lice. The mites burrow through the skin, forming small, raised, red bumps. Itching is noted and is most intense at night. Scabies can affect skin folds, even those with few hairs, such as the folds of the wrists, elbows, or between the fingers or toes.

These types of infestation are killed by medications called "pediculocides," which include the following:

- Nix™ lotion (1 percent permethrin)
- RID shampoo (pyrethrin)
- Kwell shampoo (lindane)
- Malathion 5 percent in isopropanol

Nix lotion (permethrin) will kill both the lice and their eggs. RID shampoo will kill the lice, but not their eggs. Be certain to repeat the shampoo treatment seven days later. This may not be a bad strategy with the lotion, as well. Ask your physician for a prescription for Kwell shampoo to stockpile. It is a much stronger treatment for resistant cases. It may cause neurological side effects in children, so avoid using this medicine on them. Use these products as follows:

1. Start with dry hair. If you use hair conditioners, stop for a few days before using the medicine. This will enable the medicine to have the most effect on the hair shaft.
2. Apply the medicine to the hair and scalp.
3. Rinse off after 10 minutes or so.
4. Check for lice and nits in 8–12 hours.

5. Repeat the process in 7 days.
6. Wash all linens that you don't throw away in hot water (at least 120 degrees). Unwashable items, such as stuffed animals, that you cannot bring yourself to throw out should be placed in plastic bags for 2–5 weeks (to kill off any remaining head and body lice), then opened to air outside. Combs and brushes should be placed in alcohol or very hot water. Clothes should be changed frequently, if possible.

Natural remedies for lice have existed for thousands of years. Even commercial medications such as RID shampoo use pyrethrin, which is extracted from the chrysanthemum flower. Another favorite antilice product is ClearLice™, a natural product containing peppermint, among other things, and is thought by many to be superior to standard treatments.

Another good treatment for lice is a combination of tea tree and neem (a tree in the mahogany family) oils. For external use only, mix a blend of salt, vinegar, tea tree oil, and neem oil and apply daily for 21 days. Alternatively, witch hazel and tea tree oil applied after showering daily for 21 days has been reported to be effective against hair lice.

A triple blend of tea tree, lavender, and neem oil applied to the pubic region for 21 days may also be effective in eliminating scabies, as might witch hazel and tea tree oil. Some have advocated bathing with ½ cup of Borax and ½ cup of hydrogen peroxide daily for 21 days.

Ticks

Ticks are not as clearly associated with poor hygiene as lice. Although they are commonly thought of as insects, they are actually arachnids like scorpions and spiders. The American dog tick carries pathogens (disease-causing organisms) for Rocky

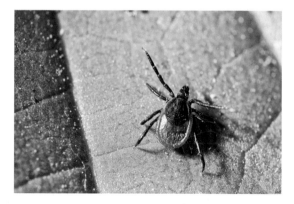

Mountain spotted fever; and the blacklegged tick, also known as the deer tick, carries the microscopic parasite that's responsible for Lyme disease. Some tick-borne illness is similar to influenza with regards to symptoms, and so is often missed by the physician. Lyme disease sometimes has a telltale "bull's-eye" rash, but other tick-related diseases may not.

Most Lyme disease is caused by the larval or juvenile stages of the deer tick. These are sometimes tough to spot because they're not much bigger than a pinhead. Each larval stage feeds only once and very slowly, usually over several days. The larval ticks are most active in summer. Although most common in the northeastern United States, they seem to be making their way farther west every year.

Ticks don't jump like fleas do; they don't fly like flies, and they don't drop from trees like your average spider. The larvae like to live in leaf litter, and they latch onto your lower leg as you pass by. Adults live in shrubs along game trails, hence the name deer tick. In inhabited areas, you might find them in woodpiles (especially in shade).

Many people don't think to protect themselves outdoors from exposure to ticks and other such potentially harmful animals, or plants, such as poison ivy. Anyone spending the day in the fresh air should take some precautions:

- Don't leave skin exposed below the knee.
- Wear thick socks (tuck your pants into them).
- Wear high-top boots.
- Use insect repellant.

A good bug repellant is going to improve your chances of avoiding bites. Citronella can be found naturally in some areas and is related to plants such as lemon grass; just rub the leaves on your skin. Oil from soybeans or eucalyptus will also work. Consider including these in your medicinal garden, if your climate is suitable.

It is important to know that the risk of contracting Lyme disease, or other tick-borne illness, increases with the length of time it feeds on someone. The good news is that there is generally no transmission of disease in the first 24 hours. The chance of infection is highest after 48 hours, so it pays to remove that tick as soon as possible. Ticks sometimes don't latch onto a person's skin for a few hours, so showering or bathing after a wilderness outing may simply wash them off. This is where good hygiene pays off.

To remove a tick, take the finest set of tweezers you have and try to grab the tick as close to the skin as you can. Pull the tick straight up; this will give you the best chance of removing it intact. If removed at an angle, the mouthparts sometimes remain in the skin, which might cause an inflammation at the site of the bite. Fortunately, it won't increase the chances of getting Lyme disease.

Afterwards, disinfect the area with Betadine or what is known as "triple antibiotic" ointment. Although other methods of tick removal, such as smothering it with petroleum jelly or lighting it on fire, are often tried, no method is more effective than pulling it out with tweezers.

Luckily, only about 20 percent of deer ticks carry Lyme or another parasitical disease. A rash that appears like a bull's-eye occurs in about half of patients. Anyone getting a rash along with flu-like symptoms that are resistant to medicines will need further treatment.

Oral antibiotics will be useful to treat early stages. Amoxicillin (500 mg 3 times a day for 14 days) or doxycycline (100 mg 2 times a day for 14 days) should work to treat the illness. These can be obtained without a prescription in certain veterinary medications (discussed later in this book). Don't be surprised if your patient still experiences muscle aches and fatigue for a time after treatment.

DENTAL CARE

Many of our readers are often surprised that a book on survival medicine devotes a portion of its pages to dental issues. History, however, tells us that problems with teeth take up a significant portion of the medic's patient load. During the Vietnam War, medical personnel noted that half of all sick call patients presented with dental complaints.

To be clear, neither of us is a dentist, and it's illegal and punishable by law to practice dentistry without a license. The lack of formal training or experience in dentistry may cause complications that are much worse than a bum tooth. If you have access to modern dental care, seek it out.

Anyone who has had to perform a task while simultaneously dealing with a bad toothache can attest to the decrease in work efficiency caused by the problem. Therefore, it only makes sense that you must learn basic dental care and procedures to handle common dental emergencies.

A survival medic's philosophy should be that an ounce of prevention is worth a pound of cure. This thinking is especially apt when it comes to your teeth. By enforcing a regimen of good dental hygiene, you will save your loved ones from a lot of pain (and yourself from a lot of headaches).

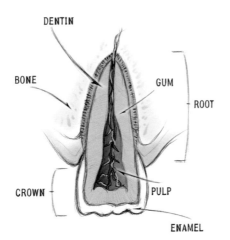

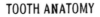

TOOTH ANATOMY

The anatomy of the tooth is relatively simple for such an important part of our body and is worth reviewing. The part of the tooth that you see above the gum line is the "crown." Below it is the "root." The bony socket that the tooth resides in is the "alveolus." Teeth are anchored to the alveolar bone with ligaments, just like you have ligaments holding together your ankle or shoulder.

The tooth is composed of several materials:

- **Enamel**—the hard, white external covering of the tooth crown
- **Dentin**—the bony yellowish material under the enamel and surrounding the pulp
- **Pulp**—connective tissue with blood vessels and nerve endings in the central portion of the tooth

Most dental disease is caused by bacteria. Your mouth is chock full of them, so anything that decreases the amount of bacteria there will reduce the chances of developing problems.

A daily brushing routine is essential, but at one point or another you will run out of toothbrushes. As an alternative, you can use your finger with a little toothpaste in a circular motion. A piece of cloth can also be used for this purpose.

Another option is to chew on the end of a twig until it gets fibrous and use that to clean your teeth. Any bendable twig (that is, live wood) will serve the purpose. This twig can serve dual purposes in that you could use the other end as a toothpick.

At one point or another, commercially made toothpaste will no longer be available. Consider baking soda as an inexpensive alternative. It's less abrasive to dental enamel than manufactured silica-based toothpaste.

Every time you eat a meal and, especially, before going to bed, you should brush your teeth or at least rinse your mouth. This will decrease inflammation in the gums and the risk of infection.

An effective and inexpensive option would be to use a solution made of ½ water and ½ hydrogen peroxide (3 percent). Swish it around in your mouth for 1–2 minutes to obtain the full effect. Most people don't include mouth rinses as part of their survival storage, but this is a great way to prevent tooth issues. Beware of higher concentrations of hydrogen peroxide, as these could burn the inside of your mouth.

Another method of preventing tooth decay is faithful flossing. It may be inconvenient for some, but a lot of bacteria accumulate between your teeth. You can prove this by flossing and then smelling the floss. Unless you're flossing regularly, it will have a foul odor due to the large amounts of bacteria you have just dislodged. Dental floss is also useful for removing foreign objects, such as food particles, from between teeth.

Tooth Decay

The stages of tooth decay

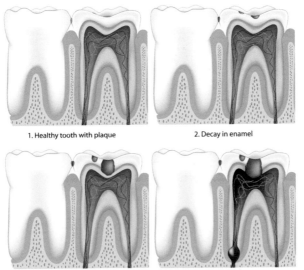

1. Healthy tooth with plaque

2. Decay in enamel

3. Decay in dentin

4. Decay in pulp

It's important to understand how bacteria causes tooth disease. Bacteria live in your mouth and colonize your teeth. Usually, they accumulate in the crevices on your molars and at the level where the teeth and gums meet. These colonies form a thick, irregular film on the base of your enamel known as tartar or plaque. The more tartar you have, the less healthy your gums and teeth are.

When you eat, these bacterial colonies also have a meal; they digest the sugars you take in and produce a toxic acid. This acid has the effect of slowly dissolving the enamel of your teeth.

Once the enamel has broken down, a "cavity" is created. When the cavity becomes deep enough to invade the soft inner part of the tooth (the pulp), the process speeds up and, because you have living nerves in each tooth, starts to cause pain. If the cavity isn't dealt with, it can lead to infection once the bacteria dig deep enough into the nerve or the surrounding gum tissue.

Inflamed gums have a distinctive appearance: They'll appear red and swollen; they'll bleed when you brush your teeth. Known as gingivitis, this is very common in adults. As the condition worsens, it can easily lead to infection. If it affects the gums, it may spread to the roots of teeth or even the bony socket.

Once the root of the tooth is involved, you could develop a particularly severe infection (abscess). This is an accumulation of pus and inflammatory fluid that causes gum swelling and can be quite painful. Once you have an abscess, you will need antibiotic therapy and, perhaps, a procedure to drain the pus that has accumulated. The tooth will likely be unsalvageable at this point.

Toothache

Treatment of a toothache starts with finding the bad tooth. Have your patient open his or her mouth so that you can investigate the area. A dental mirror and dental pick are good tools to start with. First, you will carefully look around for any obvious cavity or fracture. If there is nothing that you can see, however, you may still have serious decay between teeth or below the gums.

So how do you tell which tooth is the problem if you don't see anything obvious? Touch the teeth in the area of the toothache with something cold. The bad tooth will be very sensitive to cold. Now, touch it with something hot. If there is no sensitivity to heat, the tooth is probably salvageable.

A tooth that is probably beyond hope will cause significant pain when you touch it with something hot (only touch the tooth). It will continue to hurt for ten seconds or so after you remove the heat source. This is because the nerve has been irreversibly damaged. Once the nerve is damaged at the level of the root, you might not feel either hot or cold. It will, however, be painful to even the slightest touch.

The goal of modern dentistry is to save every tooth, if at all possible. In the old days (as recently as fifty years ago), the main treatment for a diseased tooth was extraction. In a survival setting, we may have to return to that strategy.

If you delay extracting a severely decayed tooth, it will likely get worse. Decay could spread to other teeth or cause septicemia, an infection that could spread to your bloodstream and cause major damage.

The important thing to know is this: *90 percent of all dental emergencies can be treated by extracting the tooth.*

Besides a dental pick and mirror, what else needs to be in the medic's dental kit?

Medical Dental Kit

- Dental floss, toothbrushes.
- Dental or orthodontic wax as used for braces; even a candle will do in a pinch. Wax can be used to splint a loose tooth to its neighbors.
- A rubber bite block to keep the mouth open. This will help you see the dentition and prevent yourself from getting bitten. One of those large pink erasers would serve the purpose just fine.
- Cotton pellets, Q-tips, gauze sponges (cut into small squares).
- Temporary filling material, such as Tempanol, Cavit or Dentemp™.
- Oil of cloves (eugenol), a natural anesthetic. It's important to know that eugenol burns the tongue, so never touch anything but teeth with it.
- Zinc oxide powder; mixed with two drops of clove oil, it will harden into temporary filling cement or may help fasten loose crowns.
- Dental tweezers, dental mirrors, and a dental pick.
- Extraction forceps. These are like pliers with curved ends. They come in versions specific to upper and lower teeth. Although there are many types of dental extractors, you should at least have two: number 151 or 79N for lower teeth and number 150A or 150 for upper teeth; number 23 is useful for some molar extractions.
- Elevators—one small, one medium. These are thin, chisel-like instruments that help loosen teeth by separating ligaments that hold teeth in their sockets. (Some parts of a Swiss army knife might work in a pinch.)
- A dental scaler and dental pick to remove tartar.
- Pain medication and antibiotics.

Temporary Fillings

Common dental issues will include lost fillings or loose crowns. These can be repaired, at least temporarily, by making a mixture that will harden quickly and provide a reasonable seal.

Take two drops of clove oil and mix it with zinc oxide powder to form a paste. Roll this into a ball and apply this to the area. It will harden, relieving pain at the same time.

Use your dental pick to scrape out black decay, especially at the edges of the cavity. Your paste should cover the entire area previously occupied by the original filling. Scrape off excess so that the person can close their teeth normally when they bite. You can use carbon paper or paper that you have rubbed a pencil on to identify areas where you have placed excess cement. Have your patient bite down; the carbon will stain the excess filling material dark.

It should be noted that these methods are temporary measures. Unless modern dentistry becomes available again, you will likely have to repeat the filling process multiple times.

Dental Trauma

Dental trauma may appear in various forms. After an injury to the oral cavity, a person may have any of the following:

- Dental fracture—portion of a tooth chipped or broken off
- Dental subluxation—a loose tooth
- Dental avulsion—a tooth knocked out completely

When a portion of a tooth is broken off, it is categorized on the basis of the number of layers of the tooth that are exposed. Dentists generally refer to these as Ellis class I, II, or III fractures:

Ellis I fracture: This is where only the enamel has been broken and no dentin or pulp is exposed. This is only a problem if there is a sharp edge to the tooth. You can consider filing the edge smooth or using a mixture of oil of cloves (eugenol) and zinc oxide powder as temporary cement.

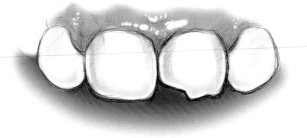

ELLIS no.1

Ellis II fracture: These fractures show yellow or beige dentin under the enamel. This area may be sensitive and should be covered if possible. The composition of dentin is different than enamel, and bacteria may enter and infect the tooth.

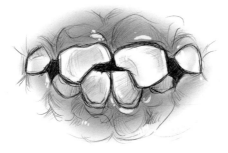

ELLIS no.2

Ellis III fracture: Here the pulp and dentin are both exposed, and Ellis III fractures can be quite uncomfortable. If the pulp is exposed, it may bleed. Protective coverings will be most necessary here, and the risks of permanent damage most likely.

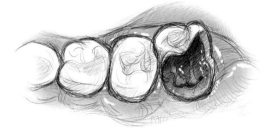

ELLIS no.3

When you identify a fracture of a tooth, you should evaluate the patient for associated damage, such as to the face, inside of the cheek, tongue, and jaw. On occasion, a tooth fragment may be lodged in the soft tissues and must be removed with instruments.

Blood is likely to be present because of the trauma, so thoroughly rinse out the inside of the mouth so you can fully assess the situation. Then, using your gloved hand or a cotton applicator, lightly touch the injured tooth to see if it is loose. Don't forget your bite block.

For sensitive Ellis II fractures of dentin, cover the exposed surface with a calcium hydroxide composition (commercially sold as Dycal™), a fluoride varnish, clear nail polish, or a medical adhesive, such as DERM-ABOND™ (medical super glue) to decrease sensitivity. Provide pain medications, and instruct the patient to avoid hot and cold food or drink.

Ellis III fractures into pulp are trouble, due to the risk of infection, among other reasons. Calcium hydroxide on the pulp surface coupled with additional temporary cement can be used as coverings. Provide analgesics and antibiotics, such as penicillin or doxycycline, are acceptable options. Despite all this, the prognosis is not favorable without modern dental intervention.

A particularly difficult dental fracture involves the root. Sometimes, it is not until the gum is peeled back that a fracture in the root is identified. If this is the case, the tooth is likely unsalvageable (especially in vertical fractures) and usually needs extraction.

Dental Subluxations and Avulsions

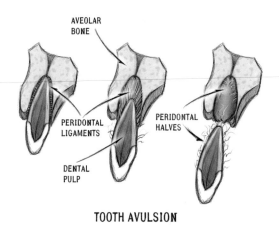

TOOTH AVULSION

A subluxation is a tooth that is knocked loose but not out of its alveolar socket. Lightly pressing the tooth with your gloved hand or a cotton applicator should identify if it is loose and how much. Minimal trauma may require no major intervention.

If a tooth is loose, it should be pressed back into the alveolus (socket) and "splinted" to neighboring teeth for stability. Dentists use wire or special materials for this purpose, but you might find yourself having to use soft wax if professional help is not at hand. If you can, use enough wax to anchor the loose tooth to neighboring teeth both in front and in back. Prevent further trauma by placing the patient on a diet of liquids and soft foods (juices, gelatin, pudding, etc.) for a time, until the tooth appears well anchored.

The most favorable situation when a tooth is completely knocked out (an avulsion) is that it came out in one piece, down to its root and ligaments. In this circumstance, time is an important factor in possible treatment success. If the tooth is not replaced or at least placed in a preservation solution, the success of reimplantation drops 1 percent every minute the tooth is not in its socket. *Note: Don't attempt to replace baby teeth.*

A good preservation liquid for teeth that have been knocked out is Hanks' solution. It helps protect raw ligament fibers for a time. This solution is available commercially as Save-a-Tooth™.

If a tooth is knocked out, do the following:

- Find the tooth.
- Pick it up by the crown, avoid touching the root, as it will damage the already damaged ligament fibers.
- Flush the tooth clean of dirt and debris with water or saline solution. Don't scrub it, as it will damage the ligament further.

If you don't have preservation solution, place the tooth in milk, saline solution, or saliva (put it between your cheek and gum, or under your tongue). This will keep your ligament cells alive longer than plain water will.

If the tooth has been out for less than 15 minutes, you may attempt to reimplant it. Flush the tooth and the empty socket with Hanks' solution (Save-a-Tooth), replace it, and cover it with cotton or gauze. Then, have the patient bite down firmly to keep it in place. Splint it with soft wax to the neighboring teeth and place your patient on a liquid diet. Antibiotics such as penicillin (veterinary equivalent: Fish Pen) or doxycycline (Bird Biotic) will be helpful to prevent infection.

You may have to soak the tooth for a half hour or so in Hanks' solution before you replace it, if it has been out for more than 15 minutes. The longer you wait to replace the tooth, the more painful it will likely be to replace, so make sure you have pain relief meds in your supplies.

After a couple of hours of being out, the ligament fibers dry out and die, and the tooth is for most intents and purposes dead. Replacing it at this point is problematic, as the pulp will decay like all dead soft tissue does. The dead tooth (which may turn dark in color) then scars down into its bony socket, acting like a dental implant. This is called "ankylosis."

It's important to know that, in mature permanent teeth, the pulp doesn't survive the injury even if the ligament does. As such, without the availability of modern dental care to remove dead tissue, even your best efforts may be unsuccessful. Serious infection in the dead pulp often ensues, and your patient may be in a worse situation than just missing a tooth.

Life with dentists may be unpleasant sometimes, but life without dentists will leave us with few options in most dental emergencies. In such circumstances, we may have to return to tooth extraction as the treatment of choice.

Dental Extraction

You, as medic, may eventually find yourself in a situation where you have to remove a diseased tooth. Tooth extraction is not an enjoyable experience as it exists today, and will be less so in a long-term survival situation with no power and limited supplies. Unlike baby teeth, a permanent tooth is unlikely to be removed simply by wiggling it out with your (gloved) hand or tying a string from it to the nearest doorknob and slamming. Knowledge of the procedure, however, will be important for anyone expecting to be the medical caregiver in the aftermath of a major disaster.

Proper positioning will help you perform the procedure more easily. The patient should be tipped at a 60-degree angle to the floor for an upper extraction (also called a maxillary extraction). The patient's mouth should be at the level of the medic's elbow. For a lower extraction (also called a mandibular extraction), the patient should be sitting upright with the mouth lower than the elbow of the medic. For right-handed medics, stand to the right of the patient; for left-handers, stand to the left. For uppers and most front lower extractions, it is best to position yourself in front of the patient. For lower molars, some prefer to position themselves behind the patient.

To begin with, wash your hands and put on gloves, a face mask, and some eye protection. You will want to keep the area around the tooth as dry as possible, so that you can see what you're doing. Some bleeding will occur, so you might want to place cotton balls or rolled gauze squares around the tooth to be removed and replace as needed.

The teeth are held in place in their sockets by ligaments, which are fibrous connective tissue. These ligaments must be severed to loosen the tooth. This is accomplished with an elevator, which looks like a small-headed flathead screwdriver or chisel.

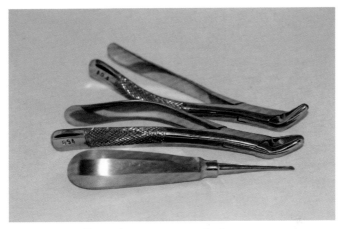

Dental extractors and elevator

Go between the tooth in question and the gum on all sides and apply a small amount of pressure to get down to the root area. This should loosen the tooth. Expect some bleeding.

Take your extraction forceps and grasp the tooth as far down the root as possible. This will give you the best chance of removing the tooth in its entirety the first time. For front teeth (which have one root), exert pressure straight downward for upper teeth and straight upward for lower teeth, after first loosening the tooth with your elevator. For teeth with more than one root, such as molars, a rocking motion will help loosen the tooth further as you extract. Once loose, avoid damage to neighboring teeth by extracting towards the cheek (or lip, for front teeth) rather than towards the tongue. This is best for all but the lower molars that are furthest back (wisdom teeth).

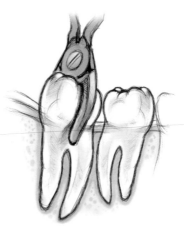

DENTAL EXTRACTOR
GRASPING ROOT

Use your other hand to support the mandible (lower jaw) in the case of lower extractions. If the tooth breaks during extraction (this is not uncommon), you will have to remove the remaining root. Use your elevator to further loosen the root and help push it outward.

Afterwards, place some gauze on the bleeding socket and have the patient bite down. A product known as ActCel hemostatic gauze is helpful to slow excessive bleeding; cut the gauze into small moistened squares and place directly on the bleeding area. It should form a gel which can be rinsed away with water in 24 hours.

Occasionally, a suture may be required if bleeding is heavy. Use 4–0 chromic catgut absorbable suture material in this case. In a recent Cuban study, what is known as veterinary "super glue" (N-butyl-2-cyanoacrylate) was used in more than one hundred patients with good success in controlling both bleeding and pain. DERMABOND glue has been used in some cases in US emergency rooms for temporary relief. Hot liquids and hard foods should be avoided for 24–72 hours.

Expect some swelling, bruising, and pain over the next few days. Cold packs will decrease swelling for the first 24–48 hours; afterwards, use warm compresses to help with jaw stiffness. Also, consider antibiotics, as infection is a possible complication. The patient should be put on a diet of liquids and soft foods to decrease trauma to the area.

Use acetaminophen (Tylenol™) or nonsteroidal anti-inflammatory medicine, such as ibuprofen, for pain (or stronger meds, if you have them). Stay away from aspirin, as it may hinder blood clotting in the socket. The blood clot is your friend, so make sure not to smoke, spit, or even use straws; the pressure effect might dislodge it, which could cause a painful condition called alveolar osteitis or "dry socket."

In this case, you will notice that the clot is gone and you may notice a foul odor in the person's breath. Antibiotics and warm saltwater gargles are useful here, and a solution of water with a small amount of clove oil may serve to decrease the pain. Don't use too much of the oil, as it could burn the mouth.

In a long-term survival situation, difficult decisions will have to be made. If modern dentistry is gone because of a mega-catastrophe, the survival medic will have to take on that role as well as that of medical caregiver. Never perform a dental procedure on someone if you have modern dental care available to you.

RESPIRATORY INFECTIONS

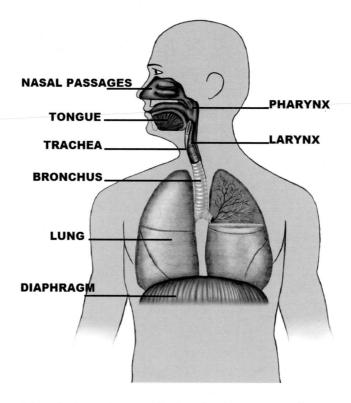

NASAL PASSAGES
PHARYNX
TONGUE
TRACHEA
LARYNX
BRONCHUS
LUNG
DIAPHRAGM

Even with today's modern medical technology, most of us can't avoid the occasional respiratory infection. Without strict adherence to sanitary protocol, it would be very easy in a major disaster for your entire community to come down with colds, sinusitis, influenza, or even pneumonia. Common colds may be caused by any of 200 different viruses. Influenza comes from viruses in the Influenza A, B, and C categories (mostly A). Over the course of history, influenza outbreaks have killed more than 100 million people.

Most of the deaths associated with influenza are not caused by the virus itself, but instead by bacterial pneumonia, a secondary infection that invades a virus-weakened immune system.

In general, most respiratory infections are spread by viral particles, and many organisms that cause these infections can live for up to 48 hours on common household surfaces, such as kitchen counters and doorknobs. Contagious viral particles can easily travel 4–6 feet when a person sneezes.

Respiratory issues are usually divided into upper and lower respiratory infections. The upper respiratory tract is considered to be anything at the level of the vocal cords (larynx) or above. The diagnosis often will be related to the affected part of the upper respiratory system. Here's how it works:

- nose—rhinitis
- throat—pharyngitis
- sinuses—sinusitis
- voice box—laryngitis
- epiglottis—epiglottitis
- tonsils—tonsillitis
- ear canal—otitis

The lower respiratory tract includes the lower windpipe, the airways (taken together, called "bronchi"), and the lungs themselves. Respiratory infections, such as bronchitis and pneumonia, are the most common cause of infectious disease in developed countries.

Symptoms of the common cold can include fever, cough, sore throat, runny nose, nasal congestion, headaches, and sneezing. Symptoms of lower respiratory infections (pneumonia and some bronchitis) include cough (with phlegm, a "productive" cough), high fever, shortness of breath, weakness, and fatigue. Most respiratory infections start showing symptoms 1–3 days after exposure to the causative organism. They can be expected to last 7–10 days if upper and somewhat longer if lower.

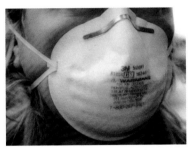

Typical N95 mask

Colds vs. Influenza

There are differences between the common cold and influenza that are helpful to know in making a diagnosis. The symptoms are similar but differ in frequency and severity. Consult the list below to identify what you're most likely dealing with:

Symptoms	Cold	Influenza
Fever	Rare, Low	Common, High
Headache	Rare	Common
Nasal congestion	Common	Occasional
Sore throat	Common	Occasional
Cough	Mild	Severe
Aches and pains	Common	Severe
Fatigue	Mild	Severe

For influenza, the administration of antiviral medications such as osel-tamivir (Tamiflu™) will shorten the course of the infection if taken in the first 48 hours after symptoms appear. After the first 48 hours, antivirals have less medicinal effect.

For colds, concentrate your treatment on the area involved: nasal congestion medication for runny noses or sore throat lozenges for pharyngitis, for example. Ibuprofen or acetaminophen will alleviate muscle aches and fevers. Steam inhalation and good hydration also give some symptomatic relief. Various natural remedies are also useful to relieve symptoms, which we discuss in the next section of this book.

Although most upper respiratory infections are caused by viruses, some sore throats may be caused by a bacterium called beta *Streptococcus* (strep throat). These patients will often have small white spots on the back of their throat, tonsils, or both and are candidates for antibiotics. Amoxicillin (veterinary equivalent: Fish Mox) or Keflex (Fish Flex) are included among the drugs of choice in those not allergic to penicillin drugs. Erythromycin (Fish Mycin) family drugs are helpful in those who are penicillin-allergic.

In most cases, however, it is not appropriate to use antibacterial agents such as antibiotics for upper respiratory infections. Antibiotics have been overused in treating these problems, and this has led to resistance on the part of some organisms to the more common drugs. Resistance has rendered some of the older antibiotics almost useless in the treatment of many illnesses.

Lower respiratory infections, such as pneumonia, are the most common cause of death from infectious disease in developed countries. These can be caused by viruses or bacteria. The more serious nature of these infections leads many practitioners to use antibiotics more often to treat the condition. Most bronchitis is caused by viruses, however, and will not be affected by antibiotics. Antibiotics may be appropriate for those with a lower respiratory infection that hasn't improved after several days of treatment with the usual medications for upper respiratory infections.

The patients who are at risk will appear to have worsening shortness of breath or thicker phlegm over the course of time despite the usual therapy.

Both upper and lower respiratory infections are different from asthma, a condition where the airways become constricted in a type of spasm when exposed to a substance. This causes a particularly vocal kind of breathing (wheeze). Asthma may occur as an allergic response, or may be associated with some respiratory infections, such as childhood "croup." The treatment of asthma involves different medicines not used with colds or flus, such as airway "openers" and epinephrine.

Good respiratory hygiene is important to prevent patients with respiratory infections from transmitting their infection to others. This is not only a good strategy for you and your family, but demonstrates social responsibility. Use the protocols below to prevent the spread of respiratory infection.

Sick individuals:

- Cover mouth and nose with tissues and dispose of those tissues safely.
- Use a mask if coughing often. Although others caring for the sick individual may wear masks (N95 masks are best for healthcare providers), it is most important for the afflicted person to wear one.
- Keep at least 4 feet away from other persons (the average distance droplets will spread), if possible.

Caregivers:

- Perform rigorous hand hygiene before and after contact. Wash soiled hands with soap and warm water for 15 seconds or clean hands with alcohol-based hand sanitizers.

- Wash down all possibly contaminated surfaces, such as kitchen counters or doorknobs, with an appropriate disinfectant (dilute bleach solution will do).
- Isolate the sick individual in a specific quarantine area, especially if he/she has a high fever.
- Wear gloves at all times when treating the patient.
- Don't self-medicate, especially with antibiotics, unless modern medical care is not accessible.

Many of the strategies and treatments described above will deal with respiratory infections quite well, but what if modern pharmaceuticals are not available or are no longer produced because of a major catastrophe? In that circumstance, we must look to our own backyard and, if we planned wisely, our medicinal garden. We will have to consider natural substances that might help alleviate various respiratory symptoms and strengthen the body's immune response.

Vitamin C, Vitamin E, and other antioxidants, taken regularly, are supposed to decrease the frequency and severity of respiratory infections. Many studies confirm their usefulness, although the duration of symptoms due to respiratory viruses per year was only decreased 1 day in one study. Despite this, antioxidant support for the immune system is important and should be part of any approach to survival food storage.

Most natural remedies are meant to target individual symptoms, such as nasal congestion or fever. There are, however, a number of alternative treatments for various respiratory infections that are reported to help stimulate the entire immune system. Consider the following essential oils:

- Geranium
- Clove Bud
- Tea tree
- Lavender

To use these oils, you would follow a procedure called direct inhalation therapy. Place 2–3 drops on the palm of your hand. Warm the oil by rubbing your hands together, and then bring your hands to your nose and mouth. Breathe 3–5 times slowly and deeply. Relax and breathe normally for two minutes, then repeat the process. Wipe any excess oil onto the throat and chest.

Many herbs may be helpful when used internally as a tea. Popular ones for general respiratory support are elderberry, *Echinacea*, licorice root, goldenseal, chamomile, peppermint, and ginseng. Antibacterial action has been also found in garlic and onion oil, fresh cinnamon, and powdered cayenne pepper. Other options include raw unprocessed honey, lemon, and apple cider vinegar, which are often added to one of the herbal teas mentioned above.

Other than general treatments, there are several good remedies to treat specific symptoms associated with colds and flu. To treat fever, for example, consider teas made from the following herbs:

- *Echinacea*
- Licorice root
- Yarrow
- Fennel
- Catnip
- Lemon balm

The underbark of willow, poplar, and aspen trees is known to be a source of salicin, the essential ingredient in aspirin. Strip off the outer bark, and take several strips of the green underbark and make a tea out of it. It should work as aspirin does to decrease fever.

To deal with the congestion that goes along with most respiratory infections, consider using direct inhalation therapy (described above) or salves with the following essential oils:

- Eucalyptus
- Rosemary
- Anise
- Peppermint
- Tea tree
- Pine
- Thyme

Another inhalation method of delivering the above herbs or even traditional medications involves the use of steam. Steam inhalation is beneficial for many respiratory ailments and is easy to implement. Just place a few drops of essential oil into steaming water and lower your face to inhale the vapors. Cover the back of your head with a towel to concentrate the steam.

Herbal teas made from the following relieve congestion:

- Stinging nettle
- Licorice root
- Peppermint
- Anise
- Cayenne pepper
- Sage
- Dandelion

Mix with honey and drink 3–4 times per day as needed. Fresh horseradish is used to open airways by taking ¼ teaspoon orally 3 times a day. Plain sterile saline solution (via nasal spray or in a "neti pot") is also used by both traditional and alternative healers.

For aches and pains due to colds, try using salves consisting of the following essential oils:

- St. John's wort
- Eucalyptus
- Camphor
- Lavender
- Peppermint
- Rosemary
- Arnica (dilute)

Teas made from the following are thought to relieve muscle ache:

- Passionflower
- Chamomile
- Valerian root
- Willow underbark
- Ginger
- Feverfew
- Rosemary

Drink the tea warm with raw honey 3–4 times a day.

For the occasional sore throat, time-honored remedies include honey and garlic "syrups," and ginger, tilden flower, or sage teas. These should be drunk warm with honey and perhaps lemon several times a day.

Gargling with warm saltwater will also bring relief. Licorice root and honey lozenges are also helpful to decrease painful swallowing.

Although the herbs described in this book have all been known to be helpful, it is important to remember that individual response to a particular herbal product differs from person to person. Also, the quality of an essential oil may differ depending on various factors, including rainfall, soil conditions, and the time of harvest.

Guide to Protective Masks

Throughout history, infectious diseases have been part and parcel of the human experience. Ever since the Middle Ages, it has been clear that some infections have the capacity of passing from person to person through the air or by contact with bodily fluids. As such, medical personnel have used masks to prevent exposure.

This makes sense from more than a selfish standpoint: In survival situations, there will be few medically trained individuals to serve a group or community. In the countries affected by the 2014 Ebola epidemic, there were only two doctors per 100,000 people. The medic, therefore, is a valuable resource. It would be a disservice to those who depend upon them if they became ill.

The basic surgical mask hasn't changed much in general appearance in the last 100 years. No doubt, you've seen photos of people wearing them in areas where there is an epidemic. In Asia, especially, it is considered socially responsible to wear them if you have a cold or flu and are going out in public. Face masks have the added advantage of reminding people to keep their hands away from their nose and mouth, a major source of the spread of infection.

If you will be taking care of your family in situations where modern medical care is unavailable, you will want a good supply of masks (and gloves) in your medical storage. Without these items, an infectious disease could possibly affect every member, including you.

Standard "medical masks" have a wide range of protection based on fit and barrier quality; three-ply masks (the most common version) are more "breathable," as you can imagine, than six-ply masks, which likely present more of a barrier. A tight fit is imperative in providing a barrier to infectious droplets.

An upgrade to the basic mask is the N95 respirator mask. N95 masks are a class of disposable respirators that have at least 95 percent efficiency against particulates larger than 0.5 microns. These are useful against many contaminants but are not 100 percent protective. There are higher level masks—N99 masks (99 percent) and N100 masks (99.7 percent)—but they are more expensive. The N stands for non-oil-resistant; there are also R95 (oil-resistant) and P95 (oil-proof) masks; these are used mostly for industrial and agricultural work.

Many of these masks have a square or round "exhalation valve" in the middle, which helps with breathability. They do not cover the eyes, however, and do not protect against gases such as chlorine. For this, you would need a "gas mask," although even these do not prevent contamination from substances absorbed through the skin.

So what would be a reasonable strategy? You'll need both standard and N95 masks as part of your medical supplies. I would recommend a significant number of each, because the masks will be contaminated once worn and should be discarded. In cases of extremely deadly diseases, such as Ebola, face shields and hoods should be added.

There are no absolute standards with regards to who wears what in the sickroom. I would recommend using the standard masks for those who are ill, to prevent contagion from coughing or sneezing (which can send air droplets several feet). Reserve the N95 masks for the caregivers. In this fashion, you will give maximum protection to those at highest risk for exposure. Remember, your highest priority is to protect yourself and the healthy members of your group. Isolate those who might be contagious, have plenty of masks, along with gloves, aprons, eye wear, and antiseptics, and pay careful attention to every aspect of hygiene.

THE EFFECTIVE SICKROOM

In normal times, we have the luxury of modern medical facilities and advanced techniques to isolate a sick patient from healthy people. If we ever find ourselves off the grid because of a disaster, most of these advantages will go the way of the dinosaur, and we will be placed in, essentially, the same medical environment we experienced in the nineteenth century.

We have the benefit, however, of knowing about sterilization and the way contagious diseases are spread, so we have a head start on our ancestors. Using this knowledge, it should be possible for the medically prepared to put together a "sickroom" or "hospital tent." This will minimize the chance of infectious diseases running rampant.

Plans for an area to care for the sick and injured should be in place whether you are at home or on the trail. If you're staying in place, designate a sickroom in your home. It should be at one end of the house, have a window or two to allow light and ventilation, and a door that can be closed. If you are in the wilderness, choose a hospital tent and place it on the periphery of your camp. Making a plan *before* a major disaster is important, as you will inevitably be kicking someone out of their room or tent if you don't. As a result, you can expect resentment at a time when everyone needs to pull together to survive.

If you don't have a spare room or tent, you'll have to erect a makeshift barrier, such as a sheet of plastic, to separate the sick from the healthy. Even if you have a dedicated sickroom, this might make sense to hang over the door as added protection. You'll want to keep those with injuries separate from those with infectious diseases, such as influenza or pneumonia, if at all possible.

Air-conditioning ducts will be close to useless in a power-down scenario, and could pose a major risk to the rest of your group. Cover them. Keep windows or vent flaps open except in particularly inclement weather to decrease the concentration of airborne pathogens.

Furnishings should be minimal, with a work surface, an exam area, and bed spaces. Cloth surfaces, such as on sofas and carpets can harbor germs and therefore should be avoided. Even bedding for the contagious might best be covered in plastic. The more areas that can be wiped down or disinfected easily, the better. (Try to do that daily with a carpet!) It's important to have a way to eliminate waste products from your bedridden patients, even if it's just a 5-gallon bucket of bleach solution. Have closed containers available for used sickroom items.

A station near the entrance of the room or tent with masks, gloves, gowns, and disinfectants would be very helpful. You'll need a basin with water, soap, or other disinfectant, and towels that should be kept for exclusive use by the caregiver. There should only be one person involved in caring for those with possibly contagious illnesses.

For supplies, get plenty of masks and gloves; gowns can be commercially made, can be plastic coveralls, or even full-body aprons. Many people consider medical supplies to consist of gauze, tourniquets, and battle dressings, but you must also dedicate sets of sheets, towels, pillows, and other items to be used in the sickroom. Keep these items separate from the bedding, bathing, and eating materials of the healthy members of your family.

Cleaning supplies should also be considered medical preparedness items. You'll want to clean the sickroom on a daily basis. Clean surfaces that may have germs on them with soap and water, or use other disinfectants. Bleach diluted in water 1:10 would be effective for this purpose. Areas to disinfect include doorknobs, tables, sinks, toilets, counters, and even toys. Wash bedsheets and towels frequently; boil them if there is no other option. Consider patient bedding and clothes to be infected, and wash or otherwise disinfect your hands right after touching them. The same goes for plates, cups, and anything else used in caring for the patient. Any medical supplies brought into the sickroom should stay there.

One additional item is important for sickroom patients: Give them a noisemaker of some sort that will enable them to alert you when they need help. This will decrease anxiety and give them confidence that you will know when they are in trouble.

FOOD-BORNE AND WATER-BORNE ILLNESS

Modern water-treatment practices and disinfectant techniques have made drinking water and eating food a lot safer than in the past. Contaminated water was the source of many deaths in olden times, and still causes epidemics of infectious disease in developing countries. It just makes common sense, therefore, that we can expect sanitation issues in the aftermath of a disaster.

Any water that has not been sterilized or any food that hasn't been properly cleaned and cooked could place an entire community at risk. As the medic, your duty will be to ensure that water is drinkable and that food-preparation areas are disinfected.

Sterilizing Water

Water can be contaminated by floods, disruptions in water service, and a number of other random events. A dead raccoon upstream from where you collect your water supplies could be a source of deadly bacteria.

Even the clearest mountain brook could be a source of parasites, called protozoa, that can cause disease. A parasite is an organism that, once it is in your body, sets up shop and causes you harm. Common parasites that cause illness include those in the *Giardia* and *Entamoeba* genera; they can affect hikers in the deepest wilderness settings.

If you're starting with cloudy water, it is because there are many small particles of debris in it. There are many excellent commercial filters of various sizes on the market that deal with this effectively. You could also make your own particulate filter by using a length of 4-inch-wide PVC pipe and inserting two or three layers of gravel, sand, zeolite, or activated charcoal, with each layer separated by pieces of cloth or cotton. Once flushed out and ready to go, you can run cloudy water through it and see clear water coming out the other side.

This type of filter, with or without activated charcoal, will get rid of particulate matter but will not kill bacteria and other pathogens. It's important to have several ways available to sterilize your water to get rid of organisms, including the following:

- **Boiling.** Use a heat source to get your water to a roiling boil. There are bacteria that may survive high heat, but they are in the minority. Using a pressure cooker would be even more thorough.
- **Chlorine.** Household bleach sold for use in laundering clothes is a 3–8 percent solution of sodium hypochlorite. Bleach has an excellent track record of eliminating bacteria, and 8–10 drops in a gallon of water will do the trick. If you're used to drinking city-treated water, you probably won't notice any difference in taste.
- **Tincture of Iodine (2 percent).** Add 12–16 drops per gallon of water. An eyedropper is useful for this purpose. You should wait 30 minutes before drinking water sterilized by iodine or bleach.
- **Ultraviolet Radiation.** Exposure to sunlight will kill bacteria! 6–8 hours in direct sunlight (even better on a reflective surface) will do the trick. Fill your clear gallon bottle and shake vigorously for 20 seconds. The oxygen released from the water molecules will help the process along and even improves the taste.

Sterilizing Food

Anyone who has eaten food that has been left out for too long has probably experienced an occasion when they have regretted it. Properly cleaning food and food-preparation surfaces is a key to preventing disease.

Your hands are a food-preparation surface. Wash your hands thoroughly before preparing your food. Other food-preparation surfaces, such as countertops, cutting boards, dishes, and utensils, should also be cleaned with water and soap or a dilute bleach solution before using them. Soap may not kill all germs, but it helps to dislodge them from surfaces.

Wash your fruits and vegetables under running water before eating them. Food that comes from plants grown in soil may have disease-causing organisms, and that's without taking into account fertilizers, such as manure. You're not protected if the fruit has a rind; the organisms on the rind will get on your hand and will be transferred to the fruit once you peel it.

Raw meats are notorious for having their juices contaminate food. Prepare meats separately from your fruits and vegetables. Ensure that meats reach an appropriate safe temperature and remain consistently at that temperature until cooked, which varies by the type of meat.

A meat thermometer is useful in ensuring this. Below is the safe cooking temperature for various meats.

Beef:	145 degrees
Pork:	150 degrees
Lamb:	160 degrees
Poultry:	165 degrees
Ground meats:	160 degrees
Sauces and gravy:	165 degrees
Soups with meat:	165 degrees
Fish:	145 degrees

DIARRHEAL DISEASE AND DEHYDRATION

With worsening sanitation and hygiene, there will likely be an increase in infectious disease, none of which will be more common than diarrhea. Diarrhea is defined as an increased frequency of loose bowel movements. If a person has three liquid stools in a row, it is a red flag that tells you to watch for signs of dehydration. Dehydration is the loss of water from the body. If severe, it can cause a series of chemical imbalances that can be life-threatening.

Diarrhea is a common ailment that may go away on its own simply by restricting your patient to clear fluids and avoiding solid food for 12 hours. However, the following symptoms that may present in association with diarrhea can be a sign of something more serious:

- Fever equal to or greater than 101 degrees
- Blood or mucus in the stool
- Black or grey-white stool
- Severe vomiting
- Major abdominal distension and pain
- Moderate to severe dehydration
- Diarrhea lasting more than 3 days

All of these symptoms may be signs of serious infection, intestinal bleeding, liver dysfunction, or even conditions that require surgery, such as appendicitis. These symptoms will also increase the likelihood that the person affected won't be able to regulate his or her fluid balance.

Epidemics caused by organisms that cause diarrhea have been a part of the human experience since before recorded history. Cholera is one particularly dangerous disease that was epidemic in the past and may be once again in the uncertain future. This infection will produce a profuse watery diarrhea with abdominal pain.

Typhoid fever is another very dangerous illness caused by contaminated food or drink. It is characterized by bloody diarrhea and pain and, like cholera, has been the cause of deadly outbreaks over the centuries. In typhoid cases, fever rises daily and, after a week or more, you may see a splotchy rash and spontaneous nosebleeds. The patient's condition deteriorates from there.

The end result (and most common cause of death) of untreated diarrheal illness is dehydration. By weight, the body is 75 percent water;

the average adult requires 2–3 liters of fluid per day to remain in balance. Children become dehydrated more easily than adults: 4 million children die every year in underdeveloped countries from dehydration due to diarrhea and other causes.

Rehydration

Fluid replacement is the treatment for dehydration. Oral rehydration is the first line of treatment, but if this fails, fluid introduced intravenously may be needed, which requires special equipment and skills. Always start by giving your patient small amounts of clear fluids. Clear fluids are easier for the body to absorb; examples include water, clear broth, gelatin, Gatorade™, and Pedialyte™.

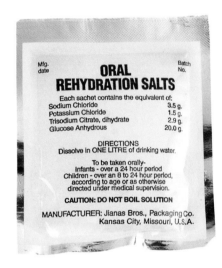

Oral rehydration packets are commercially available, but you can produce your own homemade rehydration fluid very easily: Add the following to 1 liter of water:

   6–8 teaspoons of sugar (sucrose)
   1 teaspoon of salt (sodium chloride)
   ½ teaspoon of salt substitute (potassium chloride)
   A pinch of baking soda (sodium bicarbonate)

For children, use 2 liters of water.

As the patient shows an ability to tolerate these fluids, advance the diet to juices, puddings and thin cereals, such as grits or cream of wheat. It is wise to avoid milk, as some people are lactose intolerant. Once the patient can keep down thin cereals, you may start giving them solid food.

A popular strategy for rapid recovery from dehydration is the BRAT diet, used commonly in children. This diet consists of the following:

Bananas
Rice
Applesauce
Toast (plain, or crackers)

The advantage of this strategy is that these food items are bland and easily tolerated. They also slow down intestinal motility (the rapidity of movement of food and fluids through your system), which in turn slows down water loss.

Of course, there are medicines that can help. Pepto-Bismol™ and Imodium (loperamide) will help diarrhea. They don't cure infections, but they will slow down the number of bowel movements and conserve water. These are over-the-counter medicines, and are easy to obtain. In tablet form, they will last for years if properly stored.

A good prescription medicine for vomiting is Zofran™ (ondansetron). Doctors will usually have no qualms about writing this prescription, especially for patients traveling out of the country. Of course, ibuprofen or acetaminophen is good to treat fevers. The higher the fever, the more water is lost. Therefore, anything that reduces fever will help a person's hydration status.

Various natural substances have been reported to be helpful in these situations. Herbal remedies include the following:

- Blackberry leaf
- Raspberry leaf
- Peppermint

Make a tea with the leaves and drink a cup every 2–3 hours.

Half a clove of crushed garlic and 1 teaspoon of raw honey 4 times a day is thought to exert an antibacterial effect in some cases of diarrhea. Ginger tea is a time-honored method of decreasing abdominal cramps.

As a last resort to treat dehydration from diarrhea (especially if there is also a high fever), you can try antibiotics or antiparasitic drugs. Ciprofloxacin, doxycycline and metronidazole are good choices, twice a day, until the stools are less watery. Some of these are available in veterinary form without a prescription (discussed later in this book). These medicines should be used only as a last resort, as the main side effect is usually . . . diarrhea.

IV.

✚ ✚ ✚

INFECTIONS

In the last section, we discussed infections that usually come as a result of poor sanitation and hygiene, such as diarrheal disease and body lice. There are many other types of bacterial, viral, and parasitic disease that may not necessarily have sanitation and hygiene as a factor but can be as dangerous. Appendicitis, for example, can occur in anyone, regardless of their cleanliness or the conditions at their retreat. A simple ingrown hair may lead to a boil or abscess.

Our bodies' natural ability to fight illness is impressive. There are, however, no organs that are immune to infections; the ability to recognize and treat these illnesses early is essential for the successful medic. In this section, we discuss some of the more common ones that you might see.

APPENDICITIS AND CONDITIONS THAT MIMIC IT

Appendicitis

There are various infections that can cause abdominal pain, some of which can be treated medically and some which are treated surgically. One relatively common issue that could be life threatening in a long-term survival situation, especially to young people, would be appendicitis. Appendicitis (inflammation of the appendix) occurs in approximately 8 out of every 100 people.

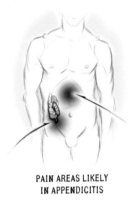

PAIN AREAS LIKELY
IN APPENDICITIS

Appendicitis can occur in anyone but most likely affects people under forty. The appendix is a tubular, worm-shaped piece of tissue 2–4 inches long that connects to the intestine at the lower right side of the abdomen. The inside of this structure forms a pouch that opens to the large intestine. The purpose of the appendix is unknown, but one theory is that it is an example of a "vestigial" organ, which means that it is a useless remnant from our evolutionary past that now serves little useful purpose.

The appendix causes trouble when it is blocked or bacteria are passed along from elsewhere in the body. The bacteria can multiply and cause inflammation or infection, and even cause the appendix to fill up with pus. If the problem is not treated, the appendix can burst, spilling infected matter into the abdominal cavity. This causes peritonitis, a condition that can spread throughout the entire abdomen and become very serious. Before the development of antibiotics, it was not unusual to die from the infection.

Appendicitis starts off with vague discomfort in the area of the belly button but moves down to the lower right quadrant of the abdomen after 12–24 hours. This area, also known as "McBurney's Point," is located about two-thirds of the way down from the belly button to the top of the right pelvic bone.

Other likely symptoms may include the following:

- Nausea and vomiting
- Loss of appetite
- Fever and chills
- Abdominal swelling
- Pain worsening with coughs or walking
- Difficulty passing gas
- Constipation or diarrhea

A patient may resist using his or her legs, because that triggers movement of abdominal muscles. Nausea, vomiting, and fever are other common signs and symptoms of appendicitis.

To diagnose this condition, press down on the lower right of the abdomen. Your patient will probably find it painful. A sign of a possible ruptured appendix may be what is called "rebound tenderness." In this circumstance, pressing down will cause pain, but it will be even more painful when you *remove* your hand.

The patient should be restricted to small amounts of clear liquids as soon as you make the diagnosis. Surgical removal of the appendix is curative here but will be difficult to carry out without modern medical facilities.

If modern surgical care is unavailable, your only hope may be giving the patient antibiotics by mouth in the hope of eliminating an early infection. Of course, intravenous antibiotics, such as cefoxitin, are more effective than related oral antibiotics, such as cephalexin (veterinary equivalent: Fish Flex). Studies in the United Kingdom achieved some success using intravenous antibiotics in early (uncomplicated) cases of appendicitis.

A combination of ciprofloxacin (veterinary equivalent: Fish Cin) and metronidazole (Fish Zole) is an option if intravenous antibiotics or surgical intervention is not available. It is also acceptable in those allergic to penicillins. Recovery, although slow, may still be possible if treatment is begun early enough or the body has formed a wall around the infection.

Can surgery be performed in situations where general anesthesia is unavailable? Most surgeries can't, without risking the loss of the patient. Surgeons in developing countries, however, have done appendectomies under local anesthesia.

Before surgery is contemplated to deal with an inflamed appendix, you must be certain that you are dealing with that exact problem. Sometimes, different medical problems present with similar symptoms, and you will have to do some detective work to differentiate one from another. This is called making the "differential diagnosis."

There are various conditions that may mimic appendicitis, including those described below.

Tubal Pregnancy

In women of childbearing age, a tubal pregnancy should be ruled out. This is a condition that occurs in 1 in every 125 pregnancies. In this condition, a fertilized egg fails to implant in the normal location (the uterine wall) and implants in the fallopian tube instead. It grows in this tiny canal until it reaches a size that bursts the tube. This, oftentimes, will cause pain and internal bleeding; in the past, it was not uncommon for a tubal pregnancy to be fatal.

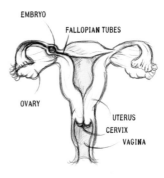

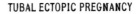

TUBAL ECTOPIC PREGNANCY

In this case, the pain is due to the presence of blood instead of an infection. If you have women of childbearing age in your family or survival group, have some pregnancy tests in your medical supplies. A woman with a missed period, positive pregnancy test, and severe pain on one side of the lower abdomen is a tubal pregnancy until proven otherwise.

Diverticulitis

Diverticulitis, unlike appendicitis, is seen mostly in older patients. Diverticula are small pouches in the large bowel that resemble an inner tube peeking out of a defect in an old-timey car tire. These areas may become blocked just as the appendix might. The symptoms are very similar, but most diverticulitis patients will complain of pain in the lower left quadrant instead of the right.

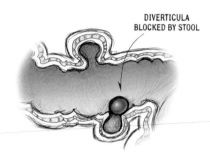

DIVERTICULA
BLOCKED BY STOOL

DIVERTICULITIS

Other inflammatory conditions in the bowel, such as Crohn's disease or ulcerative colitis, may present with pelvic pain. These are commonly treated with steroids but may require surgery, as well.

Pelvic Inflammatory Disease

A female pelvic infection often caused by sexually transmitted diseases, such as gonorrhea or chlamydia, may imitate some of the symptoms of an inflamed appendix. This is known as "pelvic inflammatory disease" (or "PID"). These patients will, however, usually have pain on *both* sides of the lower abdomen, associated with fever and, sometimes, a foul vaginal discharge.

Pelvic inflammatory disease can cause major damage to internal female anatomy. Scarring ensues as the body tries to heal, sometimes causing infertility and chronic discomfort. Serious female infections involving the pelvis are best treated with antibiotics, such as doxycycline, sometimes in combination with metronidazole twice a day for a week. It is a good idea to treat sexual partners, too.

Ovarian Cysts

Other female issues in the pelvis, such as large or ruptured ovarian cysts, could also cause pain due to pressure or bleeding. An ovarian cyst is an accumulation of fluid within an ovary that is surrounded by a wall. Many arise from egg follicles, but others can be benign or, less often, cancerous, tumors.

Most cysts cause pain by rupturing. A rupture may cause a painful irritation of the abdominal lining, internal bleeding, or both. Sometimes, ovarian cysts go away spontaneously, but a ruptured cyst that is actively bleeding will require surgery. A right-sided ruptured cyst could appear similar to appendicitis as the pain is in the same location.

The diagnosis of appendicitis or other causes of abdominal pain without modern diagnostic equipment will be challenging. Despite this, we have to remember that medical personnel, in the past, had only the physical signs and symptoms to help them reach a diagnosis.

URINARY TRACT INFECTIONS

Besides the bowels, bodily waste is excreted through the urinary tract. The urinary tract includes the kidneys, ureters, bladder, and urethra. It is, essentially, the body's plumbing.

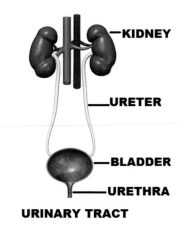

Most women, at some time of their lives, have experienced a urinary tract infection (UTI). An infection of the bladder (cystitis) usually affects the urethra (the tube that drains the bladder) as well. Various bacteria may cause this infection; *Escherichia coli* (*E. coli*) is the most common.

Although men are not immune from a bladder infection, the male urethra is much longer. Therefore, it's more difficult for bacteria to reach the bladder.

Some urinary infections are sexually transmitted, such as gonorrhea. In men, painful urination (dysuria) is very common, though most women might only note a yellowish vaginal discharge.

Although painful urination is not uncommon in cystitis, the most common symptom is frequency of the need to urinate. Some people notice that the stream of urine is somewhat hesitant ("hesitancy") or may feel an urgent need to go without warning ("urgency"). If not treated, a bladder infection may possibly ascend to the kidneys, causing an infection of those organs (pyelonephritis). Once an infection is in the kidney, your patient may experience the following symptoms:

⚕ One-sided back or flank pain
⚕ Persistent fever and chills
⚕ Abdominal pain
⚕ Bloody, cloudy, or foul urine
⚕ Dysuria
⚕ Sweating
⚕ Mental changes (in the elderly)

Antibiotics will be necessary in this instance. If the infection is not treated, the condition may progress to sepsis, where the infection reaches the bloodstream through the kidneys. These patients may show signs of shock, such as rapid breathing, decreased blood pressure, fever and chills, and confusion or loss of consciousness.

Preventative medicine plays a large role in decreasing the likelihood of this problem. Adherence to basic hygiene methods in those at high risk, especially women, is warranted. Standard recommendations include wiping from front to back after urinating or defecating, as well as urinating right after an episode of sexual intercourse. Also, never postpone urinating when there is a strong urge to do so.

Adequate fluid intake is also a key to remaining free of bladder issues. Consider natural diuretics (substances that increase urine output) to flush out your system.

Treatment revolves around the vigorous administration of fluids. Lots of water will help flush out the infection by decreasing the concentration of bacteria in the bladder or kidney. Applying warmth to the bladder region is soothing. Antibiotics are another mainstay of therapy (brand names and veterinary equivalents in parenthesis):

- Sulfamethoxazole/trimethoprim (Bactrim, Septra™; veterinary equivalent: Bird Sulfa)
- Amoxicillin (Amoxil; veterinary equivalent: Fish Mox)
- Nitrofurantoin (Macrobid™)
- Ampicillin (veterinary equivalent: Fish Cillin)
- Ciprofloxacin (Cipro™; veterinary equivalent: Fish Flox)

An over-the-counter medication that eliminates the painful urination seen in urinary infections is phenazopyridine. (Brand names include Pyridium, Uristat™, and Azo.) Don't be alarmed if your urine turns reddish-orange; it is an effect of the drug and is temporary. Vitamin C supplements are thought to reduce the concentration of bacteria in the urine.

A few natural remedies for urinary tract infections are also available:

- Garlic or garlic oil (preferably in capsules)
- *Echinacea* extract or tea
- Goldenrod tea with 1–2 tablespoons of vinegar
- Uva ursi (1 tablet)
- Cranberry juice or tablets (1–3 pills)
- Alka-Seltzer™ in 2 ounces warm water (poured directly over the urethra)

Use any of these remedies 3 times a day.

HEPATITIS

The largest internal organ in the human body is the liver. This organ is extremely important for survival, and any impairment in its function is dangerous. The liver has many duties, including the following:

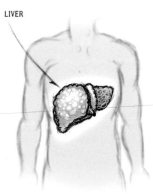

LIVER

CIRRHOSIS

- Production of bile to help digestion
- Filtration of toxins from the blood (for example, alcohol)
- Storage of certain vitamins and minerals
- Manufacture of amino acids (for protein synthesis)
- Maintenance of normal levels of glucose (sugar) in the blood
- Conversion of glucose to glycogen for storage purposes
- Production of cholesterol
- Making of urea (main component in urine)
- Processing of old red blood cells
- Development of certain hormones

Hepatitis is the term used for inflammation of the liver. Mostly caused by viruses, this condition keeps the body from being unable to process toxins and perform the other functions listed above, and can be life threatening.

There are various types of hepatitis, generally referred to by letters, such as hepatitis A, hepatitis B, and hepatitis C. Hepatitis can also occur because of adverse reactions to drugs and alcohol.

Hepatitis may also be caused by oral or fecal contamination. As such, we were in a quandary regarding whether to put this in the last section on hygiene and sanitation or here. I decided to place it here because some types of liver damage are not hygiene-related, such as those caused by alcohol abuse. Hepatitis can also be spread by sexual contact.

The hallmark of hepatitis is "jaundice," the yellowing of the skin and whites of the eyes. Urine becomes darker and stools turn grey. The liver, which can be found on the right side of the abdomen just below the lowest rib, becomes enlarged or tender to the touch. There is also a sensation of itchiness that is felt all over the body. Added to this is a feeling of extreme fatigue, weight loss, nausea, and sometimes fever. In some circumstances, people with hepatitis may have no symptoms at all and still pass the illness to others.

The hepatitis A virus is found in the bowel movements of an infected individual. When a person eats food or drinks water that is contaminated with the virus, they develop a flu-like syndrome that can quickly become serious.

Hepatitis B can be spread by exposure to infected blood, plasma, semen, and vaginal fluids. Symptoms are usually indistinguishable from hepatitis A, although they may lead to a chronic condition known as "cirrhosis," which in turn leads to permanent liver damage.

In cirrhosis, the functioning cells of the liver are replaced by nodules that do nothing to help metabolism. Cirrhosis can also be caused by long-term alcohol and chemical abuse. Possible signs and symptoms of liver cirrhosis include "ascites," an accumulation of fluid in the abdomen, varicose veins (enlarged veins, especially in the stomach and esophagus), jaundice, and swollen ankles.

About two hundred million people are chronically infected with hepatitis C virus throughout the world. It is a blood-borne virus contracted by intravenous drug use, transfusion, and unsafe sexual or medical practices. A percentage of these patients will progress to cirrhosis over time.

Other than making your patient comfortable, there isn't very much that you will be able to do in an austere setting regarding this condition. Most cases of hepatitis, however, are self-limited, which means that they will resolve on their own after a period of time. Expect at least 2–6 weeks of down time. There is a vaccine available for hepatitis B.

You can, however, practice good preventive medicine by encouraging the following policies for your family or community:

- Wash hands after using the bathroom and before preparing food.
- Wash dishes with soap in hot water.
- Avoid eating or drinking anything that may not be properly cooked or filtered.
- Make sure children don't put objects in their mouths.

There are a few "detoxifying" and anti-inflammatory herbal remedies that may help support a liver inflicted with hepatitis. Some of these supplements include the following:

- Milk thistle
- Artichoke
- Dandelion
- Turmeric
- Licorice
- Red clover
- Green tea

These are not cures but may assist your other efforts by having a restorative effect.

There are also nutritional strategies that may help:

- Avoid fatty foods and alcohol.
- Increase zinc intake.
- Decrease protein intake.
- Improve hydration status, especially with herbal teas, vegetable broths, and diluted vegetable juices.

FUNGAL INFECTIONS

Athlete's Foot

Athlete's foot (tinea pedis) is an infection of the skin caused by a type of fungus. This condition may be a chronic issue, lasting for years if not treated. Although usually seen between the toes, you might see it also on other parts of the feet or even on the hands (often between fingers). It should be noted that this problem is contagious, passed by sharing shoes or socks and even by wet surfaces.

Any fungal infection is made worse by moist conditions. People who are prone to athlete's foot commonly

- Spend long hours in closed shoes.
- Keep their feet wet for prolonged periods.
- Have had a tendency to get cuts on feet and hands.
- Perspire a lot.

To make the diagnosis, look for

- Flaking of skin between the toes or fingers.
- Itching and burning of affected areas.
- Reddened skin.
- Discolored nails.
- Fluid drainage from surfaces traumatized by repeated scratching.

If the condition is mild, keeping your feet clean and dry may be enough to enable slow improvement of the condition. However, topical antifungal ointments or powders, such as miconazole or clotrimazole, often are required for elimination of the condition.

A favorite home remedy for athlete's foot involves adding a liberal amount of tea tree oil to a foot bath and soaking for 20 minutes or so. Dry the feet well and then apply a few drops onto the affected area. Repeat this process 2 times a day. Try to keep the area as dry as possible between treatments.

Ringworm

Ringworm represents a fungal infection on the surface of the skin. It will often appear as a raised, itchy patch that is darker on the outside. As such, it may resemble a sharply-defined ring. Ringworm has nothing to do with worms.

If ringworm occurs in a hairy area, it will likely cause bald patches. Consistent scratching at the patches will cause blistering and oozing. Treatment, both conventional and natural, follows a similar process as that described for athlete's foot:

- Keep skin as dry as possible.
- Use an antifungal (miconazole, clotrimazole) or drying powders or creams.
- Avoid tight-fitting clothing on irritated areas.
- Wash regularly.
- Wash sheets daily.

Yeast Infections

In addition to viruses and bacteria, our body may be susceptible to yeast, a one-celled fungus that reproduces by budding off the parent. The human body naturally harbors certain types but can be damaged by others.

Fungal infections may be local, as in vaginal infections, "ringworm," or "athlete's foot," or they can be systemic (throughout the entire body). Some people are affected by intestinal fungal infections that can affect digestion. Systemic fungal infections have been blamed for many illnesses, but proven cases seem to occur mostly in the very young, the elderly, and those with compromised immune systems.

Vaginal Yeast Infections

Vaginal yeast infections (also called monilia) are extremely common and are not an indication of a sexually transmitted disease. A woman with a yeast infection will have a thick, white discharge reminiscent of cottage cheese and vaginal itchiness.

This infection is often easily treated with short courses of over-the-counter creams or vaginal suppositories, such as Monistat™ (miconazole), but may recur. Resistant infections may be treated with prescription fluconazole (Diflucan™) 150 mg orally once; repeat in 3 days if symptoms persist.

Nonyeast vaginal infections, those caused by bacteria or protozoa, also exist and are called bacterial vaginosis and trichomoniasis respectively. These tend to have a foul odor and are treated with the prescription antibiotic and antiparasitic metronidazole (veterinary equivalent: Fish Zole), which is taken orally.

The time-honored vinegar and water douche, performed 1 time a day, is very effective in eliminating minor vaginal infections.

Douche with 1 tablespoon of vinegar in 1 quart of water. Use this method only until your patient feels better. Women who douche often are, paradoxically, more likely to get yeast infections.

Acidophilus supplements, in powder or capsule form, may be a good oral treatment. Cranberry juice and yogurt are good foods for vaginal infections because they change the pH of the organ to a level inhospitable to yeast.

Oral Yeast Infections

A related yeast infection may be seen in the mouth of some infants and others. This infection is known as "thrush" and is identified by white patches on the inside of the cheeks, the roof of the mouth, and other areas of the oral cavity. Thrush can cause irritation, and the white patches are adherent, causing bleeding if wiped off. Occasionally, nipple tissue is affected in breastfeeding mothers.

Oral thrush may be treated conventionally with liquid fluconazole (Diflucan) 1 time a day for 1 week. Nystatin, another antifungal, is available as a "swish-and-swallow" version for oral thrush or can be applied topically 4 times a day to infected nipples for 5–7 days.

CELLULITIS

Any soft-tissue injury carries a risk of infection. Infections from minor wounds or insect bites are relatively easy to treat today, because of the wide availability of antibiotics.

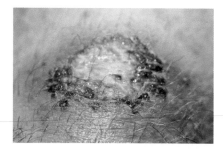

Despite your best efforts to care for a wound, there is always a chance that an infection will occur. Celluli-tis is an infection in the soft tissues below the superficial level of the skin. Below the epidermis are the main layers of soft tissue, the dermis (you've seen this area when you scraped your knee as a kid), subcutaneous fat, and muscle layers.

Although preventable, the sheer number of cuts, scrapes, and burns will make cellulitis one of the most prevalent medical problems. This infection can easily reach the bloodstream, and, without antibiotics, can cause sepsis, a life-threatening condition. Cuts, bites, blisters, or cracks in the skin can all be entryways for bacteria to cause infections that could lead to sepsis if not treated. We believe that cellulitis will be the cause of many otherwise-preventable deaths in an off-grid scenario. Conditions that might cause cellulitis include the following:

- Cracks or peeling skin between the toes
- Poor circulation, including varicose veins
- Injuries that cause a break in the skin
- Insect bites and stings, animal bites, or human bites
- Ulcers from chronic illness, such as diabetes
- Use of steroids or other medications that affect the immune system
- Wounds from previous surgery
- Intravenous drug use

The symptoms and signs of cellulitis are as follows:

- Discomfort or pain in the area of infection
- Fever and chills
- Exhaustion
- General ill feeling (malaise)

- ☤ Muscle aches (myalgia)
- ☤ Warmth in the area of the infection
- ☤ Drainage of pus or cloudy fluid from the area of the infection
- ☤ Redness, usually spreading towards torso
- ☤ Swelling in the area of infection (causing a sensation of tightness)
- ☤ Foul odor coming from the area of infection

Although the body can sometimes resolve cellulitis on its own, treatment usually includes the use of antibiotics. These can be topical, oral or intravenous. Most cellulitis will improve and disappear after a 10–14-day course of therapy with medications in the penicillin, erythromycin, or cephalosporin (Keflex) families. Amoxicillin and ampicillin are particularly popular. If cellulitis is in an extremity, keeping the limb elevated is helpful.

Acetaminophen (Tylenol) or ibuprofen (Advil) is useful to decrease discomfort. Warm-water soaks have been used for many years for symptomatic relief. The full 10–14 days of antibiotics should be completed to prevent any recurrences.

Abscesses (Boils)

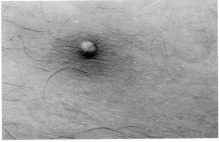

An abscess is a form of cellulitis that is, essentially, a pocket of pus. Pus is the debris left over from your body's attempt to eliminate an infection; it consists of white and red blood cells, live and dead bacteria, and inflammatory fluid.

If the abscess was not caused by an infected wound or diseased tooth, it is possible that it originated in a "cyst," a hollow structure filled with fluid. There are various types of cysts that can become infected and form abscesses:

Sebaceous–skin glands that are often associated with hair follicles and concentrated on the face and trunk.
Inclusion–where the skin lining is trapped in deeper layers as a result of trauma. Inclusions continue to produce skin cells and grow.
Pilonidal–cysts located over the area of the tailbone, which are easily infected.

Abscesses have a tendency to wall off infections; this makes it hard for antibiotics used for cellulitis to penetrate effectively. Intervention may be necessary.

To deal with an abscess, an opening must be made for the evacuation of pus. The easiest way to facilitate this is to place warm moist compresses over the area. This will help bring the infection to the surface of the skin, where it will form a "head" and perhaps drain spontaneously. This is called "ripening" the abscess. The abscess will go from firm to soft, and have a "whitehead" pimple at the point of exit.

If this fails to happen by itself over a few days, you may have to open the boil by a procedure called "incision and drainage." Using the tip of a scalpel (a number 11 blade is best), pierce the skin over the abscess where it is closest to the surface. The pus should drain freely, and your patient will probably experience immediate relief from the release of pressure.

Finally, wash thoroughly and apply some triple antibiotic ointment to the skin surrounding the incision. Cover with a clean bandage. Alternatives to triple antibiotic ointment include lavender oil, tea tree oil, and raw honey.

Incision and drainage may be helpful for dental abscesses as well but may not save overlying teeth. (See how to extract a tooth in the dental section of this book.)

Tetanus

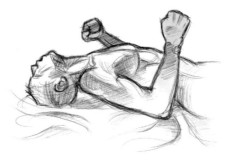

TETANUS

Classic position associated with tetanus

Most of us have dutifully gone to get a tetanus shot when we stepped on a rusty nail, but few have any real concept of what tetanus is and why it is dangerous.

Tetanus is an infection caused by the bacterium *Clostridium tetani*. The bacteria produces spores (a reproductive cell, or inactive bacteria-to-be) that primarily live in the soil or the feces of animals. These spores are capable of living for years and are resistant to extremes in temperature.

Tetanus is relatively rare in the United States, with about 50 reported cases a year. Worldwide, however, there are more than 500,000 cases a year. Most victims are found in developing countries that have poor immunization programs.

Tetanus infections usually occur when a person has experienced a break in the skin. The skin is an important barrier to infection, and any chink in the armor leaves a person open to infection. The most common cause is some type of puncture wound, such as an insect or animal bite, a splinter, or even that rusty nail. This is because the tetanus bacterium doesn't like oxygen, and deep, narrow wounds give less access to it. Any injury that compromises the skin, however, is eligible: Burns, crush injuries, and lacerations can be entryways for tetanus bacteria.

When a wound becomes contaminated with tetanus spores, the spores become activated as full-fledged bacteria and reproduce rapidly. Damage to the victim comes as a result of a strong toxin excreted by the organism, tetanospasmin. This toxin specifically targets nerves that serve muscle tissue.

Tetanospasmin binds to motor nerves, causing "misfires" that lead to involuntary contraction of the affected areas. This neural damage can be localized or affect the entire body. The patient may exhibit the classical symptom of "lockjaw," where the jaw muscle is taut. However, any muscle group is susceptible if affected by the toxin, including the respiratory musculature, which can inhibit normal breathing and become life threatening.

The most severe cases seem to occur at extremes of age, with newborns and people older than 65 most likely to succumb to the disease. Death rates from generalized tetanus hover around 25–50 percent, higher in newborns.

You will be on the lookout for the following early symptoms:

- Sore muscles (especially near the site of injury)
- Weakness

- Irritability
- Difficulty swallowing
- Lockjaw

Initial symptoms may not present themselves for up to 2 weeks. As the disease progresses, you may see the following:

- Progressively worsening muscle spasms (may start locally and become generalized over time)
- Involuntary arching of the back (sometimes so strong that bones may break or dislocations may occur)
- Fever
- Respiratory distress
- High blood pressure
- Irregular heartbeats

The first thing that the survival medic should understand is that, although an infectious disease, Tetanus is not contagious. You can feel confident treating a tetanus victim safely, as long as you wear gloves and observe standard clean technique. Wash the wound thoroughly with soap and water, using an irrigation syringe to flush out any debris. This should limit growth of the bacteria and, as a result, decrease toxin production.

You will want to administer antibiotics to kill off the rest of the bacteria in the system. Administering 500 mg of metronidazole (veterinary equivalent: Fish Zole) 2 times a day or 100 mg of doxycycline (veterinary equivalent: Bird Biotic) 2 times a day is known to be effective. The earlier you begin antibiotic therapy, the fewer toxins will be produced. Intravenous rehydration, if you have the ability to administer it, is also helpful. The patient will be more comfortable in an environment with dim lights and reduced noise.

Ventilators, tetanus antitoxin, and muscle relaxants or sedatives, such as Valium™ (diazepam), are used to treat severe cases but will be unlikely to be available to you. For this reason, it is extraordinarily important to watch anyone who has sustained a wound for the early symptoms listed above.

Tetanus can be prevented by vaccination. Booster injections are usually given every ten years. Tetanus vaccine is not without its risks, but severe complications, such as seizures or brain damage, occur in less than one in a million cases. Milder side effects, such as fatigue, fever, nausea and vomiting, headache, and inflammation in the injection site, are more common.

MOSQUITO-BORNE ILLNESSES

Mosquito bites are common vectors (transmitters) of various infectious diseases. Anaphylaxis (severe allergic reaction) as seen with bee stings is rarely an issue with mosquitos and is covered later in this book. Only female mosquitos bite humans.

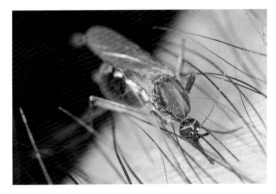

The increased amount of time we would spend outside in a survival situation would increase the chances of exposure to one or more mosquito-borne illnesses. One of the most notorious diseases caused by mosquito vectors is malaria.

Malaria is caused by a microscopic organism called a protozoan. When mosquitos bite you, they inject these microbes into your system. Once in the body, the protozoa colonize your liver. From there, they go to your blood cells and other organs.

Symptoms of malaria appear flu-like, and classically present as periodic chills, fever, and sweats. The patient becomes anemic as more blood cells are damaged by the protozoa. With time, periods between episodes become shorter and permanent organ damage may occur.

Anyone that experiences periodic fevers with severe chills and sweating should be considered candidates for treatment. Medications used for malaria include chloroquine, quinine, and quinidine.

Sometimes an antibiotic, such as doxycycline or clindamycin, is used in combination with the medications mentioned above. Physicians are usually sympathetic towards prescribing these medications to those who are contemplating trips to places where mosquitos are rampant.

Other mosquito-borne diseases include yellow fever, dengue fever, and West Nile virus. The fewer mosquitos near your retreat, the less likely you will fall victim to one of these diseases. You can decrease the population of mosquitos in your area and improve the likelihood of preventing illness by taking the following precautions:

- Look for areas of standing water that could serve as mosquito breeding grounds. Drain all water that you do not depend upon for survival.
- Repair any holes or defects in the screens on your retreat windows and doors.
- Be careful to avoid outside activities at dusk or dawn. This is the time that mosquitos are most active.
- Wear long pants and shirts whenever you venture outside.
- Have a good stockpile of insect repellants.

If you are reluctant to use chemical repellants, you may consider natural remedies. Plants that contain citronella may be rubbed on your skin and clothing to discourage bites.

When you use an essential oil to repel insects, reapply frequently and feel free to combine oils as needed. Besides citronella oil, you could use the following oils:

- Lemon eucalyptus
- Cinnamon
- Peppermint
- Geranium
- Clove
- Rosemary

V.

+ + +

ENVIRONMENTAL FACTORS

A creature's habitat is the place where it lives. This could be a forest, a lake, or the underside of a leaf. If you're a human being, your habitat is likely a town. When you are in an environment that is not your own, careful planning is necessary to avoid running afoul of the elements.

The focus of your medical training should be general, but also take into account the type of environment that you expect to live in if a disaster occurs. Learn how to treat the likely medical issues for the climate in which you'll find yourself.

Many aspects of climate can pose risk, especially extremes of ambient temperature. Humans are susceptible to damage as a result of being too cold or too hot. The body has various methods it uses to control its internal "core" temperature, either raising it or lowering it to appropriate levels. The body core consists of the major internal organ systems that are necessary to maintain life, such as the brain, heart, and liver. The remainder (skin, muscles, and extremities) is the periphery.

The body regulates its core temperature in various ways:

- **Vasoconstriction.** Blood vessels tighten to decrease flow to periphery, thereby decreasing heat loss.
- **Vasodilation.** Blood vessels expand to increase flow, thereby increasing heat loss.
- **Perspiration.** Sweat evaporates, causing a cooling effect.
- **Shivering.** Muscles produce heat by movements that create warmth.
- **Exertion.** Increasing work levels produce heat; decreasing work levels decrease heat.

Body temperature can also be regulated by adding or subtracting layers of clothing to match the environment.

Hypothermia is illness due to exposure to extreme cold. Hyperthermia, better known as heat exhaustion or heat stroke, is illness related to exposure to excessive heat.

Many environmental causes of illness are preventable with some planning. If you are in a hot environment, don't schedule major outdoor work sessions in the middle of the day. If you absolutely must work in the heat, provide a canopy, hats, or other protection against the sun. Be certain that everyone arrives well-hydrated and gets plenty of water throughout. Expect each person to require 1 pint of water an hour while working in the heat. Failure to take the above precautions could lead to dehydration, sunburns, and increased likelihood of work injury.

Likewise, those in cold environments should take the weather into account when planning outdoor activities in order to avoid hypothermia issues, such as frostbite. Youngsters, especially, will run out into the cold without paying much attention to dressing warmly. Adults will often ignore the wind-chill factor. Drugs and alcohol may impair judgment and precipitate a cold-related event.

Part of the healthcare provider's role is to educate each and every member of his or her family or group on proper planning for outdoor activities. Monitor weather conditions as well as the people you're sending out in the heat or cold. If you don't, your environment becomes a formidable enemy.

HEAT-RELATED EMERGENCIES

In the wilderness or after a natural disaster, you may find yourself without shelter to protect you from the elements. You are most likely to encounter hyperthermia (heat stroke), a common condition, in the heat of summer. However, even in cold weather, significant physical exertion in an overclothed and underhydrated individual could lead to significant heat-related injury.

The ill effects due to overheating are called "heat exhaustion" if mild to moderate, "heat stroke" if severe. Heat exhaustion usually does not result in permanent damage, but heat stroke does; indeed, it can permanently disable or even kill its victim. It is a medical emergency that must be diagnosed and treated promptly.

The risk of heat stroke correlates strongly to the heat index, a measurement of the effects of air temperature combined with humidity. Exposure to full sun increases the reported heat index by as much as 10–15 degrees.

Simply having muscle cramps or a fainting spell does not necessarily signify a major heat-related medical event. Heat cramps often occur in children who have been running around on a hot day. Getting them out of the sun, massaging the affected muscles, and providing hydration will usually resolve the problem.

A significant rise in the body's core temperature is required to warrant a diagnosis of heat exhaustion. As many heat-related symptoms may mimic other conditions, a thermometer of some sort should be part of your medical supplies.

In addition to muscle cramps, fainting, or both, symptoms of heat exhaustion can include the following:

- ♆ Confusion
- ♆ Rapid pulse
- ♆ Flushing
- ♆ Sweating
- ♆ Nausea and vomiting
- ♆ Headache
- ♆ Temperature elevation up to 105 degrees

If no action is taken to cool the victim, heat stroke may ensue. Heat stroke, in addition to all the possible signs and symptoms of heat exhaustion, can include the following symptoms:

- Loss of consciousness
- Seizures
- Bleeding (seen in the urine or vomit)
- Rapid and shallow breathing

If not dealt with quickly, shock and organ malfunction may ensue, leading to your patient's demise. The skin is likely to be hot to the touch but dry; sweating might be absent. The body makes efforts to cool itself down until it hits a temperature of 106 degrees or so. At that point, thermoregulation breaks down and the body's ability to use sweating as a natural temperature regulator fails. In heat stroke, the body core can rise to 110 degrees or more.

You'll notice that the skin becomes red, not because it is burned but because the blood vessels are dilating in an effort to dissipate some of the heat.

In some circumstances, the patient's skin may actually seem cool. It is important to realize that it is the body *core* temperature that is elevated. A person in shock may feel cold and clammy to the touch. This finding could mislead you, but simply taking a reading with your thermometer will reveal the patient's true status.

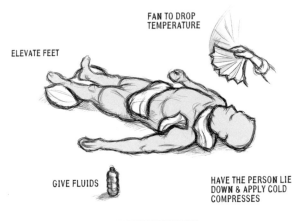

FAN TO DROP TEMPERATURE

ELEVATE FEET

GIVE FLUIDS

HAVE THE PERSON LIE DOWN & APPLY COLD COMPRESSES

HYPERTHERMIA

Treat people suspected as having hyperthermia as follows:

- Get them out of the sun or other heat source.
- Remove their clothing.
- Drench them with cool water (and ice, if available).
- Elevate their legs 12 inches above the level of their heart (the position for treating shock).
- Fan or otherwise ventilate them to help with heat evaporation.
- Place moist cold compresses on the their neck, armpits, and groin.

Why the neck, armpit, and groin? Major blood vessels pass close to the skin in these areas, and you will more efficiently cool the body core if you apply cold compresses there. In the wilderness, immersion in a cold stream may be all you have in terms of a cooling strategy. This is a worthwhile option as long as you are closely monitoring your patient.

Oral rehydration is useful to replace fluids lost, but *only* if the patient is awake and alert. Patients who are altered in mental status might "swallow" the fluid into their airways, which causes damage to the lungs.

You might think that acetaminophen or ibuprofen could help to lower temperatures, but this is actually not the case. These medications are meant to lower fevers caused by an infection, and they don't work as well if the fever was not caused by one.

Wear clothing appropriate for the weather. Tightly swaddling an infant with blankets is a recipe for disaster in hot weather. Have everyone wear a head covering. A bandanna soaked in water, for example, would be effective against the heat. Much of the sweating we do comes from our face and head, so towel off frequently to aid in heat evaporation.

If you can avoid dehydration, you will likely avoid heat exhaustion or heat stroke. Work or exercise in hot weather (especially by someone in poor physical condition) will easily cause a person to lose body water content and become dehydrated. Carefully planning your outdoor work in the summer heat and keeping up with fluids is a major step in keeping healthy and avoiding heat-related illness.

COLD-RELATED MEDICAL ISSUES

Hypothermia

Hypothermia is a condition in which body-core temperature drops below the temperature necessary for normal body function and metabolism, which is 97.5–99.5 degrees.

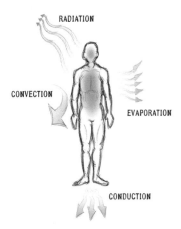

RADIATION

CONVECTION

EVAPORATION

CONDUCTION

HOW THE BODY LOSES HEAT

The body loses heat in various ways:

- **Evaporation.** The body perspires (sweats), and as the perspiration evaporates, it cools the body.
- **Radiation.** The body loses heat to the environment anytime that the ambient (surrounding) temperature is below the core temperature. For example, you lose more heat if exposed to an outside temperature of 20 degrees than if exposed to 80 degrees.
- **Conduction.** The body loses heat when its surface is in direct contact with cold temperatures, as in the case of someone falling from a boat into frigid water. Water, being denser than air, removes heat from the body much faster.
- **Convection.** Convection is a form of heat transfer where, for instance, a cooler object is in motion against the body core. The air next to the skin is heated and then removed, which requires the body to use energy to reheat. Wind chill is one example of

air convection: If the ambient temperature is 32 degrees, but the wind chill factor is at 5 degrees, you lose heat from your body as if the ambient temperature were actually 5 degrees.

The body, once it is exposed to cold, kicks into action to produce heat. The main mechanism to produce heat is shivering. Muscles shiver to produce heat, and this will be the first symptom you're likely to see of hypothermia. As the condition worsens, more symptoms will become apparent if the patient is not warmed.

Aside from shivering, the most noticeable symptoms of hypothermia will be related to mental status: confusion, lack of coordination, and lethargy. As the condition worsens, speech may become slurred; the patient will appear apathetic and uninterested in helping themselves, or may fall asleep. This occurs because of the effect of cooling temperatures on the brain: the colder the body core gets, the slower the brain works. Brain function ceases at about 68 degrees, although I have read of exceptional cases in which people (usually children) have survived even lower temperatures.

Preventing hypothermia means anticipating weather conditions you may encounter and dressing appropriately. It may be useful to remember the simple acronym COLD, which stands for cover, overexertion, layering, and dry:

Cover. Protect your head by wearing a hat. This will prevent body heat from escaping. Instead of using gloves to cover your hands, use mittens. Mittens are more helpful than gloves because they keep your fingers in contact with one another. This conserves heat.

Overexertion. Avoid activities that cause you to sweat a lot. Cold weather causes you to lose body heat quickly, and wet, sweaty clothing accelerates the process. Use regular rest periods to self-assess for cold-related changes. Pay careful attention to the status of your elderly, juvenile, or diabetic group members.

Layering. Loose-fitting, lightweight clothing in layers insulates you well. Use clothing made of tightly woven, water-repellent material for protection against the wind. Wool or silk inner layers hold body heat better than cotton does. Some synthetic materials also work well.

Dry. Keep as dry as you can. Get out of wet clothing as soon as possible. It's very easy for snow to get into gloves and boots, so pay particular attention to your hands and feet.

Travelers should anticipate the climate they will be traveling through, including wind conditions and wet weather. They should condition themselves physically to be fit for the challenge, travel with a partner, if at all possible, and have enough food and water available for the entire trip.

One factor that most people don't take into account is the effect consumption of alcohol can have in cold conditions. While it may give you a "warm" feeling, alcohol actually causes your blood vessels to expand, resulting in more-rapid heat loss from the surface of your body. The body reacts to cold by constricting the blood vessels, so expansion would negate the body's efforts to stay warm. Alcohol also causes impaired judgment, which, for example, might cause those under the influence to choose clothing that would not protect them in cold weather. This also goes for various "recreational" drugs.

If you encounter a person in a cold environment who is unconscious, confused or lethargic, you should always assume they are hypothermic until proven otherwise.

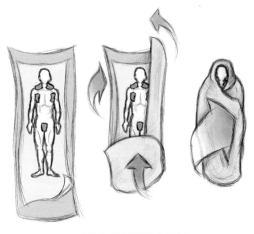

HYPOTHERMIA WRAP

Immediate action must be taken to reverse the ill effects of hypothermia. Make sure to do the following:

Get the person out of the cold. If you're unable to move the person, shield them from the cold and wind as much as possible.

Take off wet clothing. If the person is wearing wet clothing, remove them gently. Cover them with layers of dry blankets, including the head (leave the face clear). If you are outside, cover the ground to eliminate exposure to the cold surface.

Monitor breathing. A person with severe hypothermia may be unconscious. Verify that the patient is breathing and check for a pulse. Begin CPR if necessary.

Share body heat. To warm the person's body, remove your clothing and lie next to the person, making skin-to-skin contact. Then cover both of your bodies with blankets. Some people may cringe at this notion, but it's important to remember that you are trying to save a life. Gentle massage or rubbing may be helpful.

Give warm fluids orally. If the affected person is alert and able to swallow, provide a warm, nonalcoholic, noncaffeinated beverage to help warm the body.

Use warm, dry compresses. Use a dry warm compress and apply only to the neck, chest wall or groin. These areas will spread the heat much better than putting warm compresses on the extremities, which sometimes worsens the condition.

Avoid applying direct heat. Don't use hot water, a heating pad or a heating lamp to warm the person. The extreme heat can damage the skin and causes strain on the heart.

If left untreated, hypothermia leads to complete failure of various organ systems and to death. People who develop hypothermia because of exposure to cold are also vulnerable to other cold-related injuries, such as frostbite and immersion foot.

Frostbite and Immersion (Trench) Foot

Frostbite, or the freezing of body tissues, usually occurs in the extremities and sometimes the ears and nose. Initial symptoms include a "pins and needles" sensation and numbness. Skin color changes from red to white to blue. If the color then changes to black, gangrene has set in. Gangrene is the death of tissue resulting from loss of circulation. This usually results in the loss of the body part affected.

Immersion foot (formerly known as "trench foot") causes damage to nerves and small blood vessels from prolonged immersion in water. This condition appears similar to frostbite but might make the affected foot look more swollen.

Frostbite or immersion foot is treated with a warm-water (no more than 104 degrees) soak of the affected extremity. When treating these conditions, keep in mind the following:

Don't allow thawed tissue to freeze again. The more often tissue freezes and thaws, the deeper the damage. If you can't prevent your patient from being exposed to freezing temperatures again, you should wait before treating, but not more than a day.

Don't rub or massage frostbitten tissue. Rubbing frostbitten tissue will result in damage to already-injured tissue.

Don't use heat lamps or fires to treat frostbite. People with frostbite are numb and cannot feel the frostbitten tissue. Significant burns can ensue.

You can use body heat to thaw mild frostbite. You can put mildly frostbitten fingers under your arm, for example, to warm them up.

Cold Water Safety

Water doesn't have to be cold to cause hypothermia. Any water that's cooler than normal body temperature will cause heat loss. You could die of hypothermia off a tropical coast if immersed long enough. Two common situations where death from exposure occurs is when a boat capsizes or someone falls through ice.

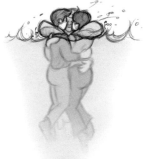

THE HUDDLE

Anyone traveling in a boat should do the following to protect against hypothermia in the event the boat capsizes:

Wear a life jacket. It can help you stay alive longer by enabling you to float without using a lot of energy and by providing some insulation. The life jackets with built-in whistles are best, so you can signal that you're in distress.

Keep your clothes on. While you're in the water, don't remove your clothing. Button or zip up. Cover your head if at all possible. The layer of water between your clothing and your body is slightly warmer and will help insulate you from the cold. Remove your clothing only after you're safely out of the water, and then do whatever you can to get dry and warm.

Get out of the water, even if only partially. The less percentage of your body exposed to cold, the less heat you will lose. Climbing onto a floating object will increase your chances of survival, even if you can only get part of your body out of the water. However, don't use up energy swimming unless you have a dry place to swim to.

Position your body to lessen heat loss. Use the heat escape lessening position (HELP) to reduce heat loss while you wait for help to arrive. Just hold your knees to your chest; this will help protect your torso (the body core) from heat loss.

Huddle together. If you've fallen into cold water with others, keep warm by facing each other in a tight circle and holding on to each other.

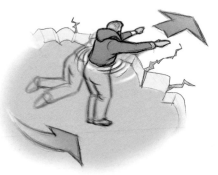

FALL THROUGH THE ICE

What if you're hiking in the wilderness and what looks like a snow field turns out to be the icy surface of a lake? Whenever you're out in the wild, it makes sense to take a change of clothes in a waterproof container so you'll have something dry to wear if you get wet. Also have a fire starter that will work even when wet.

You may be able to identify weak areas in the ice. If a thin area of ice on a lake is covered with snow, it tends to look darker than the surrounding area. Interestingly, thin areas of bare ice without snow appear lighter. Beware of areas of contrasting color as you're walking.

Your body will react to a sudden immersion in cold water by an increased pulse rate, blood pressure, and respirations. It is important to do the following:

1. Keep calm. You have some time before you succumb to the cold.
2. Breathe in and bend backward to get your head out of the water.
3. Tread water and remove objects that weigh you down.
4. Turn in the direction you came from. The ice was strong enough there.
5. Spread your arms widely on the ice.
6. Kick your feet to get momentum, and try to lift a leg up onto the ice.
7. Once on the ice, roll in the direction you came from. Do not stand up!

By rolling, you are spreading your weight out, instead of concentrating it on your feet. Crawl away until you're safe, and then work to get warm immediately.

ALTITUDE SICKNESS

In any survival situation, we might find ourselves having to relocate from a home at sea level to a retreat in the mountains. When this becomes necessary, it's likely that you will be moving fast. The rapid change in elevation will, for some, cause altitude sickness, also known as "acute mountain sickness" (AMS). This condition occurs as a result of entering an area with lower oxygen availability and reduced air pressures without first acclimating oneself.

AMS occurs most commonly at elevations approaching 8,000 feet above sea level, and is aggravated by exertion. Although it is usually a temporary condition, some patients may develop complications in the form of "edema" of certain organs. Edema is the accumulation of fluid; in altitude sickness, it may occur in the lungs (pulmonary edema) or brain (cerebral edema). Either of these conditions can be life threatening.

Like many illnesses, the best strategy against AMS is prevention. Choose the route to your retreat so that the ascent is as gradual as possible. Do not attempt more than 2,000 feet of ascent per day. Ensure that your people do not overexert themselves as they ascend, and provide lots of fresh water. Avoid the consumption of alcohol on the way.

Some normal people may be susceptible to AMS at lower elevations than others. If you have no choice but to make a rapid ascent, you should closely monitor every member of your party. Patients will usually present with symptoms similar to a hangover. If mild, they commonly include the following:

- Fatigue
- Insomnia
- Dizziness
- Headaches
- Nausea and vomiting
- Lack of appetite
- Tachycardia (fast heart rate)
- "Pins and needles" sensations
- Shortness of breath

In severe cases, you may see the following:

- Severe shortness of breath
- Confusion
- Cough and chest congestion (not nasal)
- Cyanosis (blue or gray appearance of the skin, especially the fingertips and lips)
- Loss of coordination
- Dehydration
- Hemoptysis (coughing up blood)
- Loss of consciousness
- Fever (rare)

Treating AMS first requires rest, if only to stop further ascent and allow more time to acclimate. If available, a portable oxygen tank will be useful upon onset of symptoms. A diet high in carbohydrates is thought to reduce ill effects.

A medication commonly used for both prevention and treatment of AMS is acetazolamide (Diamox™). It has a diuretic effect, which means that it speeds the elimination of excess fluid from the body by urination. Usual dosages of acetazolamide are 125–1,000 mg a day, usually starting 2 days before the planned ascent.

In normal times, you should notify your physician that you are planning a trip into high elevations and would like to avoid altitude sickness. Usually, you will be given an acetazolamide prescription in case of emergency.

There is some evidence that gingko giloba may be helpful in the natural prevention of altitude sickness. A small amount of an extract of this substance has been shown to enable the brain to tolerate lower oxygen levels. For centuries, Native Americans have benefited from using gingko for AMS.

WILDFIRE PREPAREDNESS

Fire is one of nature's ways to renew the land. Some seeds, such as those of the lodge pole pine, actually require fire to help them germinate. Despite the long-term beneficial effect to the forest, fire is an issue that presents a danger to the humans in it. Although wildfires may occur at any time of year, summertime in drought-prone areas is a particularly dangerous time.

One relevant strategy is vegetation management. Your goal is to direct fires away from your shelter, and there are a few ways to do this:

- Clear dead wood lying near your retreat. Keep woodpiles and sheds away from structures.
- Consider removing living vegetation from around your home. This might mean that you'd have to remove those thorny bushes you've planted under your windows for defense purposes.
- Have a shelter made of fire-resistant materials. A wood-frame home with wooden shingles will go up like a match in a wildfire.

So, let's create a defensible space—an area around a structure where wood and vegetation are treated, cleared, or reduced to slow the spread of wild-fire towards a structure. Having a defensible space will also provide room to work for those fighting the fire.

The amount of defensible space you'll need depends on whether you're on flat land or on a steep slope. Flatland fires spread more slowly than a fire on a slope. (Hot air and flames rise.) A fire on a steep slope with wind blowing uphill will spread quickly and produces spot fires—small fires that ignite vegetation ahead of the main burn because of small bits of burning debris in the air.

You'll want to thin out thick-canopied trees near your house. This means any nearby tree within 50 feet on flat land or 200 feet if downhill from your retreat. Prune branches off below 10–12 feet high; trees should be separated by 10–20 feet. Also eliminate all shrubs at the base of the trunks.

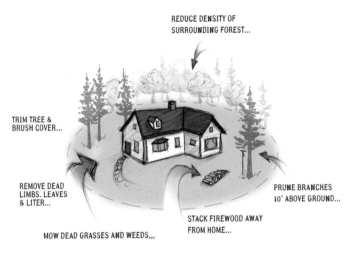

REDUCE DENSITY OF
SURROUNDING FOREST...

TRIM TREE &
BRUSH COVER...

REMOVE DEAD
LIMBS. LEAVES
& LITER...

PRUNE BRANCHES
10' ABOVE GROUND...

STACK FIREWOOD AWAY
FROM HOME...

MOW DEAD GRASSES AND WEEDS,,,

WILD FIRE SAFETY

Of course, once you have a defensible space, the natural inclination is to want to defend it, even against a forest fire. Unfortunately, you have to remember that you'll be in the middle of a lot of heat and smoke. This would make it difficult unless you're in full fire protection gear. The safest option, if there's a way out, would be to leave.

If you're leaving, have your supplies already in the car, as well as any important papers you might need to keep and some cash. If you have electricity, make sure you shut off any air-conditioning system that draws air into the house from outside. Turn off all appliances, close all windows, and lock all doors. Let others know where you're going.

If there is any possibility that you might find yourself trapped in a fire, dress in long pants, a long-sleeved shirt, and heavy boots. A wool blanket is very helpful as an additional outside layer because wool is relatively fire resistant.

If you're in a building, stay on the side of the building farthest from the fire outside. Choose a room with the least number of windows. (Windows transfer heat to the inside.) Stay there unless you have to leave because of smoke or the building's catching fire.

If that's the case, wrap yourself in that blanket, leaving only your eyes uncovered. Some people think it's a good idea to wet the blanket first.

ULTIMATE SURVIVAL MEDICINE

Don't. Wet materials transfer heat much faster than dry materials and will cause more severe burns.

If you're having trouble breathing because of the smoke, stay low and crawl out of the building if you have to. There's less smoke and heat the lower you go. Keep your face down towards the floor. This will protect your airway. Don't forget to have some eye wash in your supplies, as smoke irritates your eyes.

If you encounter a person who is actually on fire, you have to act quickly. In circumstances where a person's clothes are on fire, remember the old adage "stop, drop, and roll":

Stop. The victim will be panicked and likely running around trying to put out the flames. This generates wind, which will fan the flames. Stop the victim from running away.

Drop. Knock the victim to the ground. If possible, wrap them in a blanket. Heavy fabrics are best.

Roll. Roll the victim on the ground until the flames are extinguished. Immediately cool any burned areas of skin with water.

Smoke Inhalation

Other than burns, which are discussed in another part of this book, you can become seriously ill or even die simply from inhaling too much smoke. Remember, you can heal from burns on your skin, but you can't heal from burns in your lungs. Common causes of smoke inhalation injury include the following:

- **Simple combustion.** Combustion uses up oxygen near a fire and can kill a person simply from oxygen deficit, known as hypoxia. The larger the fire, the more oxygen it removes from the area, especially a closed space.
- **Carbon dioxide.** Some byproducts of smoke may not directly kill a person but could take up the space in the lungs that oxygen would ordinarily use.
- **Chemical irritants.** Many chemicals found in smoke can cause irritation injury when they come in contact with the lung.

This amounts to a burn inside the lung tissue, which causes swelling and airway obstruction. An example from World War I is chlorine gas.

- **Other asphyxiants.** Carbon Monoxide, Cyanide, and some Sulfides may interfere with the body's ability to use oxygen. Carbon Monoxide is the most common of these.

Symptoms may include the following:

- Cough
- Shortness of breath
- Hoarseness
- Upper airway spasm
- Eye irritation
- Headaches
- Pale, bluish, or even bright-red skin
- Loss of consciousness leading to coma or death

Your evaluation of the patient with smoke inhalation may show soot around the mouth, in the throat, and in nasal passages. These areas may be swollen and irritated. The victim will likely be short of breath and have a hoarse voice.

Of course, you will want to get your patient out of the smoky area and into an environment where there is clean air. You must be very careful not to put yourself in a situation where you are likely to succumb to smoke inhalation yourself. Always consider a mask before entering a conflagration to rescue a victim. Be prepared to use CPR if necessary.

It is important to have some way to deliver oxygen to your patient if needed. There are portable oxygen canisters that can get oxygen quickly into the lungs.

Don't expect a rapid recovery from significant smoke inhalation. Your patient will be short of breath with the slightest activity and will be very hoarse. These symptoms may go away with time or may be permanent disabilities.

Planning escape routes and having regular drills will enable your people to get out of dangerous situations quickly. If everyone knows what to do in advance, you will save precious time.

STORM PREPAREDNESS

There are few people who haven't been in the path of a major storm at one point or another. Most of those in the path of an oncoming storm will not have planned for its arrival. Some will even openly flaunt their disregard by seeking exposed areas. This is an instance where a lack of common sense can have dire consequences.

If you fail to plan ways to protect yourself and your family, you may find yourself having to treat significant traumatic injuries in the immediate aftermath. Loss of your shelter may expose your family to hypothermia or heat stroke. Later, flooding may contaminate your water supplies and expose you to serious infectious disease. Preparing to weather the storm safely will avoid major medical problems later on.

Tornado Preparedness

A tornado, or "twister," is a violently rotating column of air that is in contact with both the surface of the earth and the thunderstorm (sometimes called a "supercell") that spawned it. From a distance, tornadoes usually appear in the form of a dark funnel with all sorts of flying debris in and around it.

Tornadoes may have winds of up to 300 miles per hour and can travel for a number of miles before petering out. They may be accompanied by hail and will emit a roaring sound reminiscent of a passing train. It can be terrifying.

There are almost a thousand tornadoes in the United States every year, more than are reported in any other country. Most of these occur in "Tornado Alley," an area that includes Texas, Oklahoma, Missouri, Kansas, Arkansas, and neighboring states. Spring and early summer are the peak seasons.

Injuries from tornadoes usually come as a result of trauma from all the flying debris that is carried along with it. Strong winds can carry large objects and fling them around in a manner that is hard to believe. Indeed, there is a report that, in 1931, an 83-ton train was lifted and thrown 80 feet from the tracks.

Although some places may have sirens or other methods of warning of an approaching twister, it is important to have a plan for your family to weather the storm. Having a plan before a tornado approaches is the most likely way you will survive the event.

If you see a twister funnel, take shelter immediately. If your domicile is a mobile home, leave! They are especially vulnerable to damage from the winds. Get to the nearest building that has a tornado shelter; underground shelters are best.

If you live in Tornado Alley, consider putting together your own underground shelter. Unlike bunkers and other structures built for long-term protection, a tornado shelter has to provide safety for a short period of time. As such, it doesn't have to be very large; 8–10 square feet per person would be acceptable. Despite this, be sure to consider ventilation and the comfort or special needs of those using the shelter.

If you don't have a shelter, find a place where family members can gather if a tornado is headed your way. Basements, bathrooms, closets, or other inside rooms without windows are the best options. Windows can easily shatter from impact because of flying debris.

For added protection, get under a heavy object, such as a sturdy table. Covering your body with a sleeping bag or mattress will provide an additional shield. Discuss this plan of action with each and every member of your family or group in such a way that they will know this process by heart. Children should be taught where to find the medical kits and how to use a fire extinguisher. If possible, teach everyone how to safely turn off the gas and electricity.

If you're in a car and can drive to a shelter, do so. Although you may be hesitant to leave your vehicle, remember that they can be easily tossed around by high winds; you may be safer in a culvert or other area lower than the roadway.

In town, leaving the car to enter a sturdy building is appropriate. If there is no other shelter, however, staying in your car will protect you from some of the flying debris. Keep your seat belt on, put your head down below the level of the windows, and cover yourself if at all possible.

If you are on a hike and caught outside when the tornado hits, stay away from wooded areas. Torn branches and other debris become missiles, so an open field or ditch may be safer. Lying down flat in a low spot in the ground will give you some protection. Make sure to cover your head, if at all possible, even if it's just with your hands.

Hurricane Preparedness

A hurricane is a large tropical storm with winds that have reached a constant speed of 74 miles per hour or more. In the United States, hurricanes regularly ravage the Gulf of Mexico and the East Coast, causing billions of dollars of damage. Unlike tornados, which can pop up suddenly, hurricanes are first identified when they are hundreds, if not thousands, of miles away. We can watch their development and have a good idea of how much time we have to get ready.

Hurricanes are categorized on the basis of severity, using the Saffir-Simpson Hurricane Wind Scale. Higher-category storms may cause incredible damage and loss of life, such as occurred in Hurricane Katrina in 2005. You will have to put together an effective plan of action with regards to shelter, food, power, and other important issues.

You may also have to make a decision regarding evacuation. Unlike some disaster scenarios, you can actually outrun one of these storms if you get enough of a head start.

If you live on the coast or in an area that has flooding, there will be rising waters (storm surge) that might be enough of a reason to leave. The authorities will issue an evacuation order in many cases. A municipality often will assign a hurricane-resistant public building in your own community as a designated shelter.

If you choose to leave town, plan to go as far inland as possible. Hurricanes get their strength from the warm water temperatures over the tropical ocean; they lose strength quickly as they travel over land.

In any case, have your supplies ready to go. Although most people pack for seventy-two hours off the grid, that number is relatively arbitrary; be prepared to at least have a week's supply of food and drinking water, as well as clothes and medical supplies.

You should have an idea of what your home's weak spots are. Since South Florida was devastated by Hurricane Andrew in 1992, new homes there must have the strength to withstand 125 mph winds. Most homes, however, are made to handle 90 mph. (Hurricane strength is 74 mph.) If the coming storm has sustained winds greater than that, you may not be able to depend on the structural integrity of your home.

If you decide to stay, make sure you designate a safe room somewhere in the interior of the house. It should be in a part of the home most downwind from the direction of the winds. Make provisions for any animals you will be sheltering and move all outdoor furniture and potted plants either inside the house or up against the outside wall, preferably secured with chains. Put up hurricane shutters if you have them. Flying debris can turn into missiles during hurricanes.

Indoor planning is important, as well. Communications may be out in a major storm, so have a National Oceanic and Atmospheric Administration (NOAA) weather radio and lots of fresh batteries. You will likely lose power, so fill up your gas and propane tanks early in every hurricane season.

As the storm approaches, you'll want to fill up bathtubs and other containers with water. Turn your refrigerator and freezer down to their coldest settings, so that food won't spoil right away if the power fails. Make sure you know how to shut off the electricity, gas, and water, if necessary.

There's another kind of power you should be concerned about—purchasing power. In the aftermath of a storm, credit-card verification may be down; without cash, you may have no purchasing power at all.

Lost roof shingles are common after a hurricane, so have some water-proof tarps available. Repair crews are going to be busy after a major storm and might not get to you right away. In South Florida after Hurricane Wilma in 2005, there were still tarps on roofs more than a year later.

If you've hunkered down in your home during the storm, make sure that you've got books, board games, and light sources for when the power goes down. This will decrease anxiety and improve morale. Take time to discuss the coming storm in advance; this will give everyone an idea of what to expect and keep fear down to a minimum.

After the storm, inland floodwater may be polluted. Do not walk around in, drink, nor bathe in this water. Thorough sterilization is required. Do not eat food that has come in contact with floodwater; if unopened cans of food have been contaminated, wash them off with soap and hot water before opening.

Also, watch for downed power lines; they have been the cause of a number of electrocutions. You should never touch someone who has been electrocuted without first shutting off the power source; if you can't shut off the power, you will have to move the victim. Use a nonmetal object, such as a wooden broom handle or dry rope. If you don't, the current could pass through the individual's body and shock you.

EARTHQUAKE PREPAREDNESS

Hurricanes are more significant for residents of the Gulf or East Coasts of the United States, but the West Coast and even some areas of the Midwest have their own disaster to worry about—earthquakes. Some populated areas are near fault lines, a fracture in a volume of base rock. This is an area where movements, or seismic waves, release energy that can cause major surface disruptions.

The strength of an earthquake is measured using the Richter scale. Quakes less than 2.0 on the scale may occur every day, but are unlikely to be noticed by the average person. Each increase of 1.0 magnitude increases the strength by a factor of 10. The highest registered earthquake was the Great Chilean Earthquake of 1960 (9.5 on the Richter scale).

If the energy is released offshore, a tsunami (tidal wave) may develop. In Fukushima, Japan, a powerful earthquake (8.9 on the Richter scale) and tsunami wreaked havoc in 2011, causing major damage, loss of life, and meltdowns in local nuclear reactors.

A major earthquake is especially dangerous because of the lack of notice given beforehand. Make sure each member of your family knows what to do, no matter where they are when an earthquake occurs. Unless it happens in the dead of night, it's unlikely you will all be in the house together.

To be prepared, you'll need, at the very least, the following:

- Food and water
- Power sources
- Alternative shelters
- Medical supplies
- Clothing appropriate to the weather
- Fire extinguishers
- Means of communication
- Money (don't count on credit or debit cards being useful if the power's down)
- An adjustable wrench to turn off gas or water

Figure out where you'll meet in the event of tremors. Find out the school system's plan for earthquakes so you'll know where to find your kids.

It would be appropriate to, at least, have some food, liquids, and a pair of sturdy, comfortable shoes to keep in your car in an emergency.

Especially important to know is where your gas, electric, and water-main shutoffs are. Make sure that everyone has an idea of how to turn them off if there is a leak or electrical short. Know where the nearest medical facility is, but be aware that you may be on your own; medical responders are going to have their hands full and may not get to you quickly.

Look around your house for fixtures, such as chandeliers and bookcases, that might not be stable enough to withstand an earthquake. Flat-screen TVs, especially large ones, could easily topple. Be sure to check out kitchen and pantry shelves.

What should you do when the tremors start? If you're indoors, get under a table, desk, or something else solid, or get to an indoor hallway. You should stay clear of windows, shelves, and kitchen areas. While the building is shaking, don't try to run out; you could easily fall down stairs or get hit by falling debris. Some recommend standing under a doorway but it turns out that most doorways aren't any more solid than any other part of the structure.

Once the initial tremors are over, you can go outside. Once there, stay far away from power lines, chimneys, and anything else that could fall on top of you.

If you're in your automobile when the earthquake hits, get out of traffic as quickly as possible; other drivers are likely to be less level-headed than you are. Don't stop under bridges, trees, overpasses, power lines, or light posts. Don't leave your vehicle while the tremors are active.

One issue to be concerned about is gas leaks; make sure you don't use your camp stoves, lighters, or even matches until you're certain all is clear. Even a match could ignite a spark that could lead to an explosion. If you turned the gas off, you might consider letting the utility company turn it back on.

Don't count on telephone service after a natural disaster. Telephone companies only have enough lines to deal with 20 percent of total potential call volume at any one time. It's likely all lines will be occupied. Interestingly, this doesn't seem to include texts; you'll have a better chance to communicate by texting than by voice because of the wavelength used.

ALLERGIC REACTIONS AND ANAPHYLAXIS

In a survival situation, you may have to vacate your home and head to the outdoors. In the process, you may expose yourself to insect stings, poison oak and ivy, and strange food items to which you aren't accustomed. When your body reacts against a particular substance, we call it an "allergy."

Allergens are foreign substances that cause allergies. Our response to them can be negligible or it can be life threatening. Anaphylaxis (or anaphylactic shock) is a severe reaction and can affect the entire body. If severe enough, it can be fatal.

Minor and Chronic Allergies

Mild allergic reactions usually involve local itching and the development of a patchy, raised rash on the skin. These types of reactions may go away by themselves or with medications, such as diphenhydramine (Benadryl).

Chronic allergies may manifest as a skin condition, eczema. This is a red, patchy rash in different places that is itchy and flaky. This type of rash usually responds well to 1 percent hydrocortisone cream, although sometimes a stronger steroid cream, such as clobetasol (prescription) may be necessary. The very worst cases may require oral steroids, such as prednisone.

If the allergic reaction is minor, there are various essential oils you can apply to relieve symptoms such as itching:

- Peppermint
- Lavender
- Chamomile (German or Roman)
- Calendula
- Myrrh
- Cypress
- *Helichrysum*
- Wintergreen
- Eucalyptus
- Blue Tansy
- Aloe Vera

To use the above oils, you would dilute 50/50 with olive or coconut oil; apply 2 drops to the affected area daily.

Hay Fever

Hay fever, also known as allergic rhinitis or seasonal allergy, is a collection of symptoms, mostly affecting the eyes and nose, that occur when you breathe in something you are allergic to. Hay fever may be triggered by dust, animal dander, insect venom, fungi, or pollens. Sufferers of allergic rhinitis can have the following symptoms:

- Nasal congestion
- Sneezing
- Red eyes with tearing
- Itchy throat, eyes, and skin

Antihistamines, such as Claritin and Benadryl, are old standbys for this type of allergy. Alternative therapies for hay fever include essential oils for use on the skin from the following:

- German chamomile
- Roman chamomile
- Lavender
- Eucalyptus
- Ginger

Apply 2 drops to each temple, 2–4 times per day. Alternatively, add 1 drop of the oil to a bowl of steaming water, covering the head with a towel and inhale slowly for 15 minutes. A number of teas to drink that may be useful are licorice root, stinging nettle, and St. John's wort. Drink 1 cup daily 3 times a day.

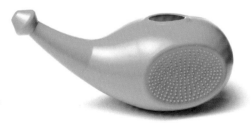

Neti pot

A neti pot is a useful item to have to deal with allergic reactions affecting the nasal passages. It looks like a small teapot. With a neti pot, you can wash out pollen and clear congestion and mucus. Use with a sterile saline (saltwater) solution daily as follows:

1. Bend over a sink.
2. Tilt your head to one side.
3. Keep your forehead and chin at the same level to keep water out of your mouth.
4. Breathe through your mouth during the procedure.
5. Insert the spout gently into your uppermost nostril.
6. Pour the solution so that it drains through the lower nostril.
7. Blow your nose to clear your nostrils.
8. Tilt your head to the other side, and repeat with the other nostril.

Recently, there have been concerns about neti pots from the FDA. They warn that the pots are meant to be used with sterilized saline; in 2011, two people lost their lives to infections after using contaminated water.

Asthma

Asthma is a chronic condition that affects your ability to breathe. It affects the airways that transport air to your lungs. When people with asthma are exposed to an allergen, these airways become inflamed and swollen. This decreases the diameter of the airway, and less air gets to the lungs. As such, you will develop shortness of breath, tightness in your chest, and start to wheeze and cough (an "asthma attack").

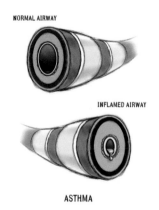

NORMAL AIRWAY

INFLAMED AIRWAY

ASTHMA

In rare situations, the airways can become so constricted that a person could suffocate from lack of oxygen. The following are some common allergens that trigger an asthma attack:

- Pet or wild animal dander
- Dust or the excrement of dust mites
- Mold and mildew
- Smoke
- Pollen
- Severe stress
- Pollutants in the air
- Some medicines

There are many myths associated with asthma, including the following:

- Asthma is contagious.
- Someone with asthma will grow out of it.
- If someone who has asthma moves to a new area, his or her asthma will go away.

And the following is true:

- Asthma may become dormant for a time, but the risk that it will return is always there.
- Asthma is hereditary. If both of a patient's parents have asthma, the patient has a 70 percent chance of developing it, compared with only 6 percent if neither parent has it.
- Asthmatic symptoms may be different from attack to attack and from individual to individual.

The following are the main symptoms of asthma:

- Cough
- Shortness of breath
- Wheezing (usually sudden)
- Chest tightness (sometimes confused with a heart attack)
- Rapid pulse rate and respiration rate
- Anxiety

Besides these main symptoms, there are others that signal a life-threatening episode. A patient with asthma who has become cyanotic—has blue/gray color to their lips, fingertips, and face—is in trouble.

In severe asthma, it takes longer to exhale than to inhale. Wheezing may take on a higher pitch. A patient who has spent too much time without adequate oxygen will become confused, then drowsy, and then possibly lose consciousness.

To make the diagnosis, use a stethoscope to listen to the lungs on both sides. Make sure that you listen closely to the bottom, middle, and top lung areas. In a mild asthmatic attack, you will hear relatively loud, musical noises when the patient breathes. As the asthma worsens, less air is passing through the airways and the pitch of the wheezes will be higher and perhaps not as loud. If no air is passing through, you may hear no sounds at all.

You can measure how open the patient's airways are with a simple diagnostic instrument, the peak-flow meter. By having a patient forcefully exhale into it, you can identify whether his or her cough is part of an asthma attack, or whether they are having a panic attack instead, which can have some of the same symptoms.

Take a baseline peak-flow measurement when the patient is well. With moderate asthma, peak flow will be reduced 20–40 percent. Greater than 50 percent is a sign of a severe episode. With a cough that is not related to asthma, or upper respiratory infection, the peak flow will be close to normal. The same goes for a panic attack; despite shortness of breath, the peak flow is still about normal.

The cornerstones of asthma treatment are avoiding allergens that trigger attacks and maintaining open airways. Medications come in one of two forms: drugs that give quick relief from an attack, and drugs that control the frequency of asthmatic episodes.

Quick-relief drugs include inhalers that open airways (known as bronchodilators), such as Albuterol (Ventolin, Proventil™). These drugs should open airways quickly and give significant relief. Don't be surprised if you notice a rapid heart rate in patients on these medications; it's a common side effect.

Patients who use quick-relief asthmatic medications more than twice a week are candidates for daily control therapy. These drugs work (when taken daily) to decrease the number of episodes and are usually some form of inhaled steroid. They may be in the form of pills or inhalers. Remember that inhalers lose potency over time. An expired inhaler, unlike many pills or tablets, will lose potency relatively quickly.

It's important to figure out what allergens trigger a patient's asthma attacks and work out a plan for avoiding them as much as possible. Furthermore, make sure to stockpile as much asthma medication as possible in case of emergency. Physicians are usually sympathetic to requests for extra prescriptions from their asthmatic patients.

Mild to moderate cases of asthma can be helped with the use of natural remedies. There are actually quite a few substances that have been reported to be helpful.

With a number of these substances, further research is needed to corroborate how much these affect severe asthma, so take standard medications if your peak flow reading is 60 percent of normal or less.

Don't underestimate the effect of your diet. To improve your diet and ease your asthma, try the following:

- Replace animal proteins with plant proteins.
- Increase intake of omega-3 fatty acids.
- Eliminate milk and other dairy products.
- Eat organically whenever possible.
- Eliminate trans fats and instead use extra-virgin olive oil as your main cooking oil.
- Always stay well-hydrated; drinking fluids will make your lung secretions less viscous.

Finally, various breathing methods, such as taught in yoga classes, are thought to help promote well-being and control the panic response seen in asthmatic attacks.

Natural Remedies for Asthma

Ginger and garlic tea. Put four minced garlic cloves in some ginger tea while it's hot. Cool it down and drink twice a day.

Other herbal teas. Ephedra, coltsfoot, codonopsis, butterbur, nettle, chamomile, turmeric, and rosemary all have the potential to improve an asthmatic attack.

Coffee. Black, unsweetened coffee is a stimulant that might make your lungs function better when you are having an attack. Don't drink more than 12 ounces at a time, as coffee can dehydrate you.

Eucalyptus. Use in a steam or direct inhalation to open airways. Rub a few drops of oil between your hands or in steaming water and breathe in deeply.

Honey. Breathing deeply from a jar of honey should improve breathing in a few minutes. To decrease the frequency of attacks, stir 1 teaspoon of honey into a 12-ounce glass of water and drink it 3 times daily.

Licorice and ginger. Mix licorice and ginger (½ teaspoon of each) in a cup of water. *Warning: Licorice can raise blood pressure.*

Mustard oil rub. Mix mustard oil with camphor and rub it on your chest and back.

Vitamin D. Some asthmatics have been diagnosed with vitamin D deficiency.

Anaphylactic Reactions

In a small percentage of people, an immune response to an allergen may affect more than just a local area. Severe allergic reactions involve various organ systems and can be quite dangerous.

Anaphylactic reactions were first identified when researchers tried to protect dogs against a certain poison by desensitizing them with small doses. Instead of being protected, many of the dogs died suddenly the second time they got the poison. They were killed by their own immune systems going out of control.

The following are proven causes of anaphylaxis:

- **Drugs**—dyes injected during x-rays, antibiotics (such as Penicillin), anesthetics, aspirin and ibuprofen, and even some heart and blood pressure medicines
- **Foods**—nuts, fruit, and seafood
- **Insect stings**—bees and yellowjacket wasps
- **Latex**—rubber gloves made of latex
- **Exercise**—often after eating
- **Idiopathic**—meaning "of unknown cause"

It's important to recognize the signs and symptoms of anaphylaxis, because the faster you treat it, the less likely it will be life threatening. They include the following:

- **Rashes.** This often occurs at places not associated with the actual exposure, for example, an all-over rash in someone with a bee sting on the arm.
- **Swelling.** This can be generalized, but sometimes isolated to the airways or throat.
- **Breathing difficulty.** Wheezing is common, as in asthmatics.
- **GI symptoms.** These can include diarrhea, nausea and vomiting, or abdominal pain.
- **Loss of consciousness.** The patient may appear to have fainted.
- **Paresthesias.** This can include strange sensations on the lips or oral cavity, especially with food allergies.
- **Shock.** Blood pressure drops, respiratory failure leading to coma and death.

Fainting is not the same thing as anaphylactic shock. You can tell the difference in several ways: Someone who has fainted is usually pale in color, but a patient in anaphylactic shock will often appear somewhat flushed. The pulse in anaphylaxis is fast, but a person who has fainted will have a slow heart rate. Most people who have just fainted will rarely have breathing problems and rashes, but these will be common signs and symptoms in an anaphylactic reaction.

With food allergies, victims may notice the effects occur very rapidly; indeed, their life may be in danger within a few minutes. People who have had a serious anaphylactic reaction should be observed overnight, as there is, on occasion, a second wave of symptoms—sometimes several hours after the exposure.

A major player in this cascade of anaphylaxis is histamine, which triggers an inflammatory response. Medications that counteract these ill effects are known, therefore, as antihistamines. These drugs may be helpful in mild allergic reactions. In tablet form, antihistamines such as diphenhydramine (Benadryl) take about an hour to get into the blood-stream properly.

In an anaphylactic reaction, this isn't fast enough to save lives. If it's all you have, chew the pill to get it into your system more quickly. It still, however, may not be enough. As such, we look to another medicine that *is* more effective: adrenaline, known in the United States as epinephrine.

Adrenaline (epinephrine) is a hormone that is produced in the adrenal glands, small organs near the kidneys. Epinephrine makes your heart pump faster, widens the air passages so you can breathe, and raises your blood pressure. The hormone works successfully against all of the effects of anaphylaxis. Therefore, it should be part of your medical supplies.

Adrenaline (epinephrine) is delivered through an injection. Inhalers have been tried in the past but have disadvantages. Anaphylactic reactions cause difficulty breathing. If you can't inhale, you won't get much benefit from an inhaler.

The EpiPen is the most popular of the various commercially available kits to combat anaphylaxis. It's important to learn how to use it properly. Here's how you do it:

1. Remove the EpiPen from its case.
2. Hold it firmly in your fist.
3. Remove the cap (some have two caps).

4. Have the patient sit or lie down.
5. Hold the thigh muscle still.
6. Press the end firmly against the thigh in a perpendicular fashion; it should click.
7. Hold for 10 seconds.
8. Massage the injection site.
9. Dispose of the needle safely.

Remember that the EpiPen won't help you if it isn't readily accessible. Any allergic members of your family or group should always have it in their possession.

Because it's a liquid, adrenaline (Epinephrine) will not stay effective forever, as some pills or capsules might. Be sure to follow the storage instructions. While the EpiPen should not be stored in a hot place, it also shouldn't be kept where it could freeze, which will damage its effectiveness significantly.

You will have limited quantities of this drug, so when do you break into those precious supplies? An easily remembered formula is the rule of D's:

Definite reaction—an obvious, major reaction, such as a large rash or difficult breathing.

Danger—any worsening of a reaction after a few minutes.

Deterioration—use the EpiPen before the condition becomes life threatening. When in doubt, use it. It's wise to have more than one handy.

An imminent danger is probably likely only if your patient has difficulty breathing or has lost consciousness. Inhalation of stomach acid into the lungs or respiratory failure is a major cause of death in these cases.

Some people may not be able to take adrenaline (epinephrine) because of chronic heart conditions or high blood pressure. Make sure that your people consult with their healthcare providers to make sure it's safe for them to use.

POISON IVY, OAK, AND SUMAC

Unless you live in Alaska, Hawaii, or the middle of the desert, the outdoors will have a population of poison ivy, poison oak, poison sumac, or all three. Once exposed to one or the other, 85 percent of the population will develop an immune response against it that will generate an itchy rash of varying degrees of severity. Winter does not eliminate the possibility of a reaction, as you

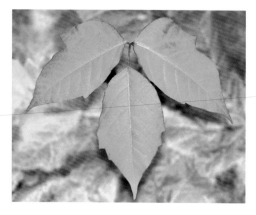

Poison ivy

can have a reaction against the urushiol (the toxic oil that causes a reaction after the first sensitizing exposure) even when vines or shrubs are dormant.

As the saying goes, "leaves of three, let it be." Although it is true that poison ivy comes in "leaves of three," so do many other plants. Familiarize yourself with what it looks like.

Poison ivy and poison oak are very similar in that they both have urushiol. Poison ivy leaves may be pointier, with poison oak often looking more like, well, oak leaves. One or both is present just about everywhere in the continental United States.

Poison sumac is a shrub or small tree, growing up to nearly 30 feet in height in parts of the eastern United States. Each leaf has 7–13 pointy leaflets. Although poison sumac has the same irritant present in poison ivy and poison oak, it is far more powerful. Simply inhaling smoke from burning poison sumac has been reported to cause death by suffocation.

All of these plants contain urushiol. The oil is in the vines, leaves, and roots. The best prevention is not allowing your skin to come in contact with the oil. If you can't avoid being close to these plants, take the following precautions:

- Wear long pants, long-sleeved shirts, work gloves, and boots in areas known to have the plants.
- Consider an over-the-counter lotion, IvyBlock™, as a preventative. Apply it as you would a sunblock to likely areas of exposure.

Theoretically, it will prevent the oil from being absorbed by your skin.

The rash takes from several hours to several days to become apparent, and will appear as red, itchy, patchy bumps. Sometimes the rash appears almost linear.

Urushiol can remain active for years, even on your clothes, so thorough laundering is necessary. Routine body washing with soap will not be useful after 30 minutes of exposure, as your system will already be producing antibodies. Hot water seems to help the oil absorb into the skin, so use only cold water early on. After all the irritant has been absorbed, however, hot water baths are recommended by some to relieve itching.

Cleansers that remove resin or oil, such as Fels-Naptha soap or Tecnu™ poison oak and ivy cleansers, are more effective than regular detergent and can be used even several hours after exposure. Rubbing alcohol is another reasonable option and easily carried as hand sanitizers or prep pads.

Even if you choose not to treat the rash, it will go away by itself in 2–3 weeks. Although it is temporary, it could be so itchy as to make you absolutely miserable. Diphenhydramine (Benadryl) at 25–50 mg dosages 4 times a day will be helpful in relieving the itching. It's important to know that the 50 mg dosage will make you drowsy. Unfortunately, calamine lotion, an old standby, and hydrocortisone cream will probably not be very effective. Some astringent solutions, such as Domeboro, have been reported to give relief from the itching.

Severe rashes have been treated with the prescription dose pack of Medrol (methylprednisolone, a drug similar to prednisone). Prednisone is a strong anti-inflammatory drug and will be more effective in preventing the inflammatory reaction that your antibodies will cause.

There are several alternative treatments for poison ivy, oak, and sumac:

- Apple cider vinegar (use to cleanse the irritated area)
- Essential oils mixed with Aloe Vera gel, such as tea tree, lemon, lavender, peppermint, geranium, and chamomile
- Baking soda paste
- Epsom salt baths
- Jewelweed (mash and apply)
- Chamomile tea bag compresses

VI.

✚ ✚ ✚

INJURIES TO SOFT TISSUES

The performance of daily survival tasks, such as chopping wood and cooking food, may lead to a number of soft-tissue injuries (those that do not involve bony structures). From a simple cut to a severe burn, any damage to skin is a hole in your body's protective armor.

Each wound is different and must be evaluated separately. If not present at the time the wound is incurred, the medic should begin by asking the simple question: "What happened?" A look around at the site of the accident will give you an idea of what type of debris you might find in the wound and the likelihood of infection. Initially, always assume a wound is dirty. Other questions to ask are whether the victim has chronic medical problems, such as diabetes, and whether they are allergic to any medications.

The physical examination of a wound requires assessing the following:

- Location on the body
- Length of the wound
- Depth of the wound
- Type of tissue involved (skin, muscle, bone)
- Circulation and nerve involvement

If the injury is in an extremity, have the patient show you a full range of motion, if possible, during your examination. This is especially important if the injury involves a joint.

This section deals with various injuries, their evaluation, and treatment.

MINOR WOUNDS

A soft-tissue injury is considered minor when it fails to penetrate the deep layer of the skin, the dermis. This would include cuts, scrapes, and bruises:

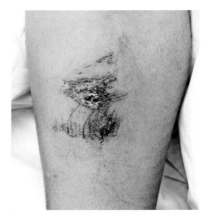

- ⚕ **Cuts and scratches.** These tears in the skin only penetrate the epidermis (superficial skin layer) and become infected on an infrequent basis in a healthy person.
- ⚕ **Abrasions.** This is where a portion of the epidermis has been scraped off. You probably have experienced plenty of these as a child.
- ⚕ **Bruises or Contusions.** These result from blunt trauma and do not penetrate the skin at all. However, there is bleeding into the skin from blood vessels that have been disrupted by the impact.

All of these minor injuries can be treated easily:

- Wash the wound thoroughly.
- Use of an antiseptic, such as Betadine; honey; or an antibiotic ointment, such as Neosporin or Bactroban™ (mupirocin) is helpful in preventing infection.
- Treat minor pain with over-the-counter drugs such as ibuprofen and acetaminophen.

Minor bleeding can be stopped with a wet styptic pencil, an item normally used for shaving cuts. If the skin is broken, the wound should have a protective adhesive bandage placed over it to prevent infection. A liquid bandage, such as New-Skin™, is an excellent way to cover a minor injury.

Applying pressure and ice (if available) wherever a bruise seems to be spreading will stop it from getting bigger. Bruises will change color over time from blackish blue to brown to yellow as they heal.

The following is an alternative process to deal with these issues:

1. Evaluate seriousness of wound; if minor, you may continue with home remedies.
2. Stop minor bleeding with herbal blood clotting agents such as yarrow, cinnamon, or cayenne pepper powder. Compress the area with gauze.
3. After minor bleeding is stopped, clean the wound with an herbal antiseptic. Mix a few drops of oil with sterile water and wash out the wound thoroughly. Essential oils with this property include:
   • Lavender oil
   • Tea tree
   • Rosemary
   • Eucalyptus
   • Peppermint
   • Other natural antiseptics, including garlic, raw unprocessed honey, *Echinacea*, witch hazel, and St. John's wort
4. Dress the wound using clean gauze. Do not wrap too tightly.
5. Change the dressing, reapply antiseptic, and observe for infection twice daily until healed.

HEMORRHAGIC AND MAJOR WOUNDS

In a major disaster, traumatic wounds may be commonplace. Therefore, the medic for a family or group must be prepared for the worst possible injuries.

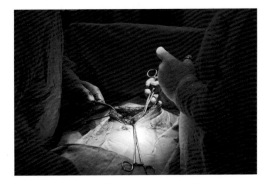

Cuts in the skin can be minor or catastrophic, superficial or deep, clean or infected. Most significant cuts (also called lacerations) penetrate both the dermis and epidermis and are associated with bleeding, sometimes major. Bleeding can be venous in origin, which manifests as dark red blood, draining steadily from the wound. Bleeding can also be arterial, which is bright red (because of the higher oxygen content) and comes out in spurts that correspond to the pulse of the patient. As the vein and artery usually run together, a serious cut can have both.

Once below the level of the skin, large blood vessels, tendons, and nerves may be involved. Assess circulation, sensation, and the ability to move the injured area. Vessel and nerve damage are more likely to occur in deep lacerations and crush injuries.

For an extremity injury, evaluate the capillary refill time to test for circulation beyond the area of the wound. To do this, press the nail bed, or finger or toe pad; with a person with normal circulation, this area will turn white when you release pressure and then return to a normal color within two seconds. If it takes longer or the fingertips are blue, there may be a damaged blood vessel. If sensation is decreased (test by lightly pricking with a safety pin beyond the level of the wound), there may be nerve damage.

Evaluating Blood Loss

Evaluating blood loss is an important aspect of dealing with wounds. An average-size human adult has about 10 pints of blood. The effect on the body caused by blood loss varies with the amount of blood loss incurred:

- **1.5 pints (0.75 liters) or less.** The patient experiences little or no effect. You can donate 1 pint of whole blood, for example, as often as every 8 weeks.
- **1.5–3.5 pints (0.75–1.5 liters).** Rapid heartbeat and respiration occurs. The skin becomes cool and may appear pale. The patient is usually very agitated. If you are not accustomed to the sight of blood, you might be, too. Even a small amount of blood on the floor or on the patient may make an inexperienced medic queasy.
- **3.5–4 pints (1.5–2 liters).** Blood pressure begins to drop; the patient may appear confused. Heartbeat is usually very rapid.
- **More than 4 pints (2 liters):** The patient is now very pale, and may be unconscious. After a period of time with continued blood loss, the blood pressure drops further, the heart and respiration rates decrease, and the patient is in serious danger.

As the medic, you should always have nitrile gloves in your pack; wearing them when treating the patient will keep the wound from becoming contaminated. Try to avoid touching the palm or finger portions of the gloves as you put them on. If there are no gloves, grab a bandanna or other cloth barrier and press it onto the wound.

The cornerstone of hemorrhage control is direct pressure. This measure often will stop bleeding all by itself. Bleeding in an extremity may be slowed by elevating the limb above the level of the heart.

Pressure points are locations where major arteries come close enough to the skin to be compressed manually. Pressing on the pressure point for the area injured may help slow bleeding further down the track of the blood vessel.

Using pressure points, we can map specific areas on which to concentrate our efforts to decrease bleeding. For example, there is a large blood vessel, the popliteal artery, behind each knee. If you have a bleeding wound in the lower leg, applying pressure on the back of the knee will help stop the hemorrhage. A diagram of some major pressure points is below.

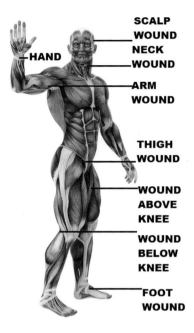

SCALP WOUND
NECK WOUND
HAND
ARM WOUND
THIGH WOUND
WOUND ABOVE KNEE
WOUND BELOW KNEE
FOOT WOUND

If this fails to stop the bleeding, it may be appropriate to use a tourniquet. Most are simple to use and could even be placed with one hand. An improvised version can be made with a folded bandanna (at least 2 inches wide) and a stick, but avoid rope or wire. Tourniquets must be placed tightly; arterial bleeding usually requires more pressure than simple venous bleeding to stop it.

The placement of a tourniquet to a wound must be made judiciously. The tourniquet stops bleeding from the open blood vessel, but it also stops circulation in nearby intact blood vessels as well. In survival settings, it is important to note that the tourniquet, once placed, should be loosened every 10 minutes or so, to enable blood flow to uninjured areas. Also, this will enable the medic to determine whether clotting has stopped the bleeding.

Tourniquets are painful if they are in place for too long, and prolonged use could actually cause the patient to lose a limb from lack of circulation. Your body may also build up toxins in the extremity; these become concentrated and rush into your body core when you release the tourniquet. It takes less than an hour or two with a tourniquet in place to cause this problem. As such, you should mark the victim with the time that the tourniquet was placed.

Once you are comfortable that major bleeding has abated, release pressure from the tourniquet but leave it in place. Irrigate (flush) the wound aggressively with sterile water or a solution of 1 part Betadine to 10 parts water. Most studies find that sterilized water is just as good as a concentrated antiseptic solution for wound healing (sometimes better). Although it is acceptable to perform a first cleaning with Betadine or hydrogen peroxide, later cleaning should definitely not use these concentrated products. New cells are trying to grow, and concentrated antiseptics dry out these fragile new cells and slow healing.

Packing the wound with bandages is not just for sopping up blood; the process helps apply pressure. It's important to make sure that you put the most pressure where the bleeding was occurring in the wound. If the blood was coming from the top of a large wound, start packing there.

Now cover the whole area with a dry dressing for further protection. The Israeli army developed an excellent bandage which is easy to use and is found almost everywhere survival gear is sold. The advantage of the Israel battle dressing is that it applies pressure on the bleeding area for you. This enables the medics to have hands free for further care, or to attend additional victims.

Bandages get dirty and should be changed often, twice a day at a minimum, until the wound has healed.

Knife and Gunshot Wounds

The process described above of stopping hemorrhage and dressing a wound will also work for traumatic injuries, such as knife and gunshot wounds. You have probably heard that you should not remove a knife because it can cause the hemorrhage to worsen. This will give you time to get the patient to the hospital, but what if there are no hospitals? You will have to transport your victim to your base camp and prepare to remove the knife. Have plenty of gauze and clotting agents available.

Bullet wounds are the opposite, in that the bullet is usually removed if at all possible when modern medical care is available. If you do not have the luxury of transferring the patient to a trauma center, you will want to avoid digging for a hard-to-find bullet. Even though there are instruments made for this purpose, manipulation could cause further bleeding and lead to infection.

For a historical example, take the case of President James Garfield. In 1881, he was shot by an assassin. In their rush to remove the bullet, twelve different physicians placed their (ungloved) hands in the wound. The wound, which would not have been mortal in all probability, became infected. As a result, the president died. In austere settings, think twice before removing a projectile that isn't clearly visible and easily reached.

Remember that the process described above is meant for survival situations where help is *not* coming.

Commercial Hemostatic Agents

In studies of battlefield casualties, 50 percent of those killed in action died of blood loss; 25 percent died within the first "golden" hour after being wounded. A victim's chance of survival diminishes significantly after 1 hour without care, with a threefold increase in mortality for every 30 minutes without care thereafter.

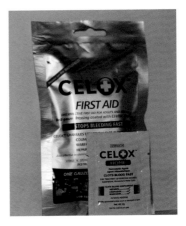

The control of major hemorrhage may be the territory of the trauma surgeon, but what if you find yourself without access to modern medical care? In the last decade or so, there have been major advancements in hemostasis (stopping blood loss).

Although there are various types of hemostatic agents on the market for medical storage, the two most popular are QuickClot and Celox. Both are available in a powder or powder-impregnated gauze.

QuickClot originally contained a volcanic mineral, zeolite, which effectively clotted bleeding wounds but also caused a reaction that caused some serious burns. The current generation is made from kaolin, a clay mineral that is the original ingredient in Kaopectate™. It does not contain animal, human, or botanical components.

One negative with QuickClot is that it does not absorb into the body and can be difficult to remove from the wound. This was certainly true of previous generations, but it is claimed no longer to be as big an issue, especially if you use the brand's gauze dressing.

Celox is the other popular hemostatic agent. It is composed of chitosan, an organic material processed from shrimp shells. Despite this, the company claims that it can be used in patients allergic to seafood. When Celox comes in contact with blood, it bonds with it to form a clot that appears as a gel. Like QuickClot, it also comes in impregnated gauze dressings.

Celox will cause effective clotting even in those on anticoagulants, such as heparin, warfarin, or Coumadin™, without further depleting clotting factors. Chitosan, being an organic material, is gradually broken down by the body's natural enzymes into other substances normally found there. Like QuickClot, Celox is FDA-approved. Studies by the US government compare Celox favorably to other hemostatic agents.

A downside to use of hemostatic agents is that they may be difficult to remove in advance of surgical intervention. As such, they are rarely used by emergency medical personnel in normal times.

Both QuickClot and Celox gauze dressings have been tested by the United States and United Kingdom militaries and have been put to good use in Iraq and Afghanistan. Although effective, these items should not be used as a first line of treatment in a bleeding patient. Pressure, elevation of a bleeding extremity above the heart, gauze packing, and tourniquets should be your strategy here. If these measures fail, however, you have an effective extra weapon to stop that hemorrhage.

Soft-Tissue Wound Care

Once you have stopped the bleeding and applied a dressing, you are in safer territory than you were. In an austere setting, however, you must follow the status of the wound until full recovery in your role as medic. An open wound can heal by two methods:

Primary Intention (Closure). The wound is closed in some way, such as with sutures or staples. This results in a smaller scar but carries the risk of inadvertently sequestering bacteria deep in the wound.

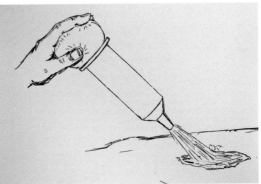

Irrigating the wound

Secondary Intention (Granulation). Leaving a wound open causes the formation of granulation tissue, rapidly growing early scar tissue that is rich in blood vessels. It fills in spaces where the wound edges are not together. After a period of time, it turns into mature scar tissue. This scar is larger than if the wound were closed by primary intention, but decreases the risk of infection if properly cared for.

Remember the old saying "The solution to pollution is dilution." Using a bulb or irrigation syringe (60–100 ml) will provide pressure to the flow of water and wash out old clots and dirt. Lightly scrub any open wound with diluted Betadine or sterilized water. You may notice some (usually slight) bleeding. This is a sign of tissue that is forming new blood vessels and not necessarily a bad sign. Apply pressure with a clean bandage until it stops.

Wound dressings must be changed regularly (at least twice a day or whenever the bandage is saturated with blood or other fluids) to give the best chance for quick healing. When you change a dressing, it is important to clean the wound area with sterilized (drinkable) water or an antiseptic solution, such as a dilute solution of 1 part Betadine to 10 parts water.

An alternative antiseptic solution that is easy to make using common storage supplies is Dakin's solution. First used during WWI, this solution is used to disinfect wounds on the skin, such as pressure sores in bedridden patients. It is inexpensive to put together, dissolves dead cells, and is composed of the following:

- Sodium hypochlorite solution (regular-strength household bleach)
- Sodium bicarbonate (baking soda)
- Boiled tap water

To make Dakin's solution, add ½ teaspoon of baking soda to 4 cups of sterilized water. Then, add bleach to reach the strength that you'll need: 3 teaspoons will act as a mild antiseptic effect (plenty for clean wounds that are healing), and 3 tablespoons will give you a stronger effect for infected wounds. Do not take Dakin's solution internally, and watch for allergic reactions in the form or rashes or other irritation. Store in darkness at room temperature and make a new batch frequently, as it loses potency quickly. Do not freeze or heat up the solution.

To ensure rapid healing of open wounds, we use a type of dressing method known as "wet-to-dry." Apply a bandage that has been soaked in sterilized water and wrung out directly to the wound. New cells are prevented from drying out by keeping them in a moist environment. On top of the bandage that touches the healing wound, place a dry bandage and some type of tape to secure it in place. Thus, you have a wet-to-dry dressing.

It may also be a good idea to apply some triple antibiotic ointment around a healing wound to prevent infection from bacteria on the skin. Raw honey, lavender oil, and tea tree oil are some natural alternatives.

As time goes on, you might see some blackish material on the wound edges. This is nonviable material and should be removed. It might just scrub out, or you may need to take your scissors or scalpel and trim off the dead tissue. Called debridement, this procedure removes material that is no longer part of the healing process.

Wound Closure

There is always some controversy as to whether to close a wound. When and why would you choose to close a wound, and what method should you use? One rule of thumb is to always use the least invasive methods first; in order, they are tapes, glues, staples, and sutures.

There are several methods available to close a laceration. It makes common sense to use the simplest and least invasive method that will do the job. The easiest to use are Steri-Strips and butterfly closures, adhesive bandages that adhere on

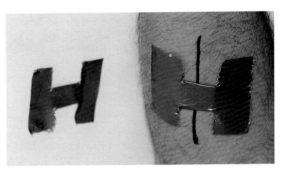

Improvised butterfly closure with duct tape

each side of the wound to pull it together. They don't require puncturing the skin and will fall off on their own, in time. Even duct tape can be used to make a butterfly closure.

The second-least-invasive method is cyanoacrylate, special glue sold as DERMABOND™. This is medical-grade adhesive made specifically for use on the skin. Simply hold the skin edges together and run a thin line of glue over the laceration. Hold in place until dry. It will naturally peel off as the skin heals.

Some have recommended (the much less expensive) household product Super Glue™ for wound closure. This preparation is slightly different chemically, and is not made for use on the skin. It may cause skin irritation in some, and burn-like reactions have been reported.

You can test Super Glue for allergic reactions by placing a small amount on the inside of your forearm and observe for a rash over the next 24 hours.

Another closure method is the use of skin staplers. They work by "pinching" the skin together and should be removed in about 7 days. You will require two toothed tweezers ("Adson forceps") to evert the skin edges and approximate them for the person doing the stapling. As such, stapling is best done if you have an assistant. The most skilled person is actually the one holding the tweezers, not the person stapling.

Staples are best removed with a specific instrument known as a staple remover. Stapling equipment is widely available but probably not as cost-effective as other methods.

Using sutures is the most invasive method of wound or laceration closure. As it can be done by a single person, it is the one that requires the most skill. Before you choose to close a wound by suturing, make sure you ask yourself why you can't use a less invasive method instead. In a long-term survival situation, it's unlikely you'll ever be able to replenish those items.

When to Close a Wound

What are you trying to accomplish by stitching a wound closed? Your goals should be simple: You close wounds to repair the defect in your body's armor and to promote healing. A well-approximated wound also has less scarring.

Unfortunately, here is where it gets complicated. Closing a wound that should be left open can do a lot more harm than good, and could possibly put your patient's life at risk. The decision to close a wound is not automatic but involves serious considerations.

The most important consideration is whether you are dealing with a clean or a dirty wound. Most wounds you will encounter in a survival setting will be dirty. If you try to close a dirty wound, you have sequestered bacteria and dirt into the body. Within a short period of time, the infected wound will become red, swollen, and hot. An abscess may form, and pus will accumulate inside.

The infection may spread to the bloodstream and, when it does, the patient's life is in danger. Leaving the wound open will enable you to clean the inside frequently and observe the healing process. It also enables inflammatory fluid to drain out of the body. Wounds that are left open heal from the inside out. The scar isn't as pretty, but it's the safest option in most cases.

Other considerations when deciding whether or not to close a wound are whether it is a simple laceration (straight, thin cut on the skin) or whether it is an avulsion (areas of skin torn out, hanging flaps). If the edges of the skin are so far apart that they cannot be stitched together without undue pressure, the wound should be left open. If the wound has been open for more than 8 hours, it should be left open; bacteria have already had a good chance to colonize the injury.

If you're certain the wound is clean, you should close it if it is long, deep, or gapes open loosely. Exceptions would include any type of animal or human bite.

Lacerations over moving parts, such as the knee joint, will be more likely to require stitches. Remember that you should close deep wounds in layers, to prevent any unapproximated "dead space" from occurring. Dead spaces are pockets of bacteria-laden air in a closed wound that may lead to a major infection.

If you are unsure, you can wait 72 hours before closing a wound to make sure that no signs of infection develop. This is referred to as "delayed closure." Some wounds can be partially closed, allowing a small open space to avoid the accumulation of inflammatory fluid. Drains, consisting of thin lengths of latex, nitrile, or even gauze may be placed into the wound for this purpose. Of course, you should place a dressing over the exposed area.

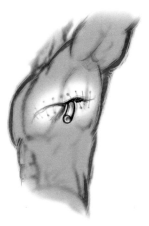

PENROSE DRAIN IN PLACE

Many injuries that require closure also should be treated with antibiotics to decrease the chance of infection. Natural remedies, such as fresh crushed garlic or raw unprocessed honey may be useful in an austere setting.

Deep-layer sutures are never removed, so try to use absorbable material, such as chromic catgut or VICRYL if possible. If you must use nonabsorbables, such as silk, nylon, or prolene, the body will wall off the sutures and may form a nodule known as a "granuloma." This may be disconcerting, but has little effect on a patient's health.

Sutures on the skin should be removed in 7 days (5 days if on the face); if over a joint, 14–21 days. Stitches placed over a joint, such as the knee, should be placed close together. In other areas, ½ inch or more between sutures is acceptable. It is alright to allow space for drainage of fluid from the wound.

For an even more in-depth discussion of suturing, stapling, and anesthetic blocks, see our comprehensive book *The Survival Medicine Handbook*.

Blisters, Splinters, and Fishhooks

Anyone who has done any hiking or has bought the wrong pair of shoes probably has experienced a friction blister. For a relatively small soft-tissue injury, it can certainly cause more than its share of problems. More than one hike has come to a screeching halt because the terrain was more than the foot-wear could handle. Never underestimate the importance of a properly fitted pair of shoes.

Each part of your foot should be comfortable in your new boots:

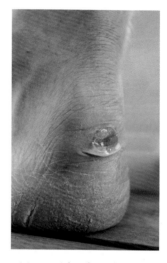

Typical broken blister

- The ball of your foot should fit the widest part of the shoe without issue.
- There should be about ½ inch or so from the end of your toes to the end of your shoe.
- The upper part of the shoe should be flexible enough to not cause discomfort on your instep.
- Your heel should not slip up and down when you walk.

Other considerations are important: Soles should be thick Vibram™ or other sturdy material. High-cut boots will help prevent ankle sprains by giving more support and will protect against snakebite.

Don't buy shoes that are too tight and expect them to stretch. They might, but you'll go through a lot of discomfort to get them there. You might be used to buying shoes online, but you really should walk in a shoe first for a while before making any purchases. Unless you can count shoemaking as one of your survival skills, buy a spare pair or two now while they're still available.

Heavier boots, such as those with steel toes, are great if you're chopping wood (you get to keep all ten of your toes) but are heavy. Remember that 1 extra pound of weight in your boot is like 5 extra pounds of weight on your back. In wet climates, waterproof materials such as Gore-Tex™, with flexible uppers, are a good investment.

Socks also factor into the health of your feet. Most people hike in the same pair of socks all day, even in the heat of summer.

Sweaty feet are unhappy feet; wetness increases friction and gives you blisters.

Change your socks often and have replacement pairs as a standard item in your backpack. Consider the use of a lighter, second pair of socks (sock liners) under the thicker hiking socks you use for additional protection. Foot powders, such as Gold Bond, or even cornstarch can help your feet stay dry.

Blisters

If a blister is just starting, it will look like a tender red area where the friction is. Cover it with moleskin or Spenco™ 2nd Skin™ before it gets worse. If you don't have any on hand, you can make use of gauze or a Band-Aid or even duct tape. The important thing here is to add padding to lessen the friction on the area.

Most people are eager to pop their blisters, but this shouldn't be done with small ones, as this could lead to infection. Large blisters are different, however. Follow this process:

1. Clean the area with disinfectant. Alcohol or iodine is especially useful.
2. Take a needle and sterilize it with alcohol or heat it until it is red hot.
3. Pierce the side of the blister. This enables the fluid to drain. This will ease some discomfort and also will enable healing to begin.
4. Preserve loose skin; cover the blister to offer protection.
5. Apply antibiotic cream if possible.
6. Take some moleskin or Spenco 2nd Skin and cut a hole in the middle a little bigger than the blister.

7. Place the moleskin on so that the blister is in the middle of the opening.
8. Cover with a gauze pad or other bandage.
9. Rest if you can.

If you absolutely must keep walking, make sure that your bandage has stopped the friction to the area. Remember, bandages frequently come off, so check it from time to time to make sure it's still on. Change the bandage frequently to maintain cleanliness.

Several home remedies can help in treating blisters:

- A cold compress to the blister by soaking a cloth in salt water.

- A 10 percent tannic-acid solution to the blister 2–3 times a day.

- A few drops of Listerine™ antiseptic to a broken blister to disinfect the wound. Garlic oil is also very useful for this purpose.

- Place some aloe vera, vitamin E oil, or zinc oxide ointment on the blister.

- Witch hazel on the blister 3 times a day to help with pain and dry it out.

- Tea tree oil to prevent infection.

Splinters

Being out in the forest or working with wood sometimes leaves a person with a splinter or two to deal with. You can remove a splinter by simply cutting the skin over it until the end can be grasped with small forceps or tweezers. You'll need a magnifying glass to make this process easier.

If you can see the entire length of the splinter, use a scalpel (number 11 or 15 blade) and cut the epidermis. You want to cut superficially and just enough to expose the tip of the wooden fragment. Then, take your tweezers and grasp the end of the splinter and pull it out along the angle that it entered the skin. Don't forget to wash the area thoroughly before and after the procedure.

It's unlikely that a major infection will come from simply having a splinter, with the exception of those that have been under the skin for more than 2–3 days. Redness or swelling in the area will become apparent if an infection is brewing. You might consider antibiotics in this circumstance to avoid having problems later.

Fishhooks

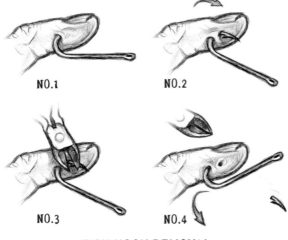

NO.1   NO.2

NO.3   NO.4

FISH HOOK REMOVAL

Even if you're an accomplished fisherman, you will eventually wind up with a fishhook embedded in you somewhere, probably your hand. Since the hook probably has worm guts on it, start off by cleaning the area thoroughly with an antiseptic.

Your hook probably has a barbed end. If you can't easily slide it out, the barb is probably the issue. Press down on the skin over where the barb is and then attempt to remove the hook along the curve of the shank.

If this doesn't work, you may have to advance the fishhook further along the skin until the barbed end comes out again. At this point, you can take a wire cutter and separate the barbed end from the shank. Then, pull the shank out from whence it came. Wash the area again and cover with a bandage. Observe carefully over time for signs of infection.

BURN INJURIES

If you find yourself off the power grid, you will be cooking out in the open more frequently. The potential for significant burn injuries will rise exponentially, especially if the survival group includes small children; naturally curious, they may get too close to your campfires. A working knowledge of burns and their treatment will be a standard skill for every group's medical provider.

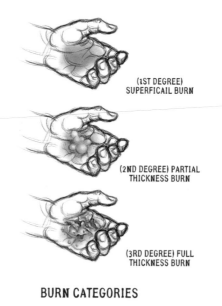

(1ST DEGREE) SUPERFICAIL BURN

(2ND DEGREE) PARTIAL THICKNESS BURN

(3RD DEGREE) FULL THICKNESS BURN

BURN CATEGORIES

The severity of the burn injury depends on the percentage of the total body surface that is burned, and on the degree (depth) of the burn injury. Although assessing the surface percentage is helpful to burn units in major hospitals, this practice will likely be of limited helpfulness in austere settings.

Before we discuss the different degrees of burn you might encounter, let's talk about prevention. Most burns you'll see will be due to too much exposure to the sun. Take the following steps to avoid sunburn:

- Stay out of the sun whenever possible.
- Avoid work during peak sun hours (say, 11 a.m.–4 p.m.).
- Wear long pants and sleeves, hats, and sunglasses.
- Spend rest periods in the shade.

If you cannot avoid extended exposure to sunlight, be certain to apply a sunblock. Do this before going outside and frequently throughout the day. Even water resistant and waterproof sunscreens should be reapplied generously every 1–2 hours.

By the way, a sunblock and a sunscreen are not the same thing. Sunblock contains tiny particles that block and reflect ultraviolet (UV) light;

sunscreen contains substances that absorb UV light, thus preventing it from penetrating the skin. Many commercial products contain both.

The SPF (sun protection factor) rating system was developed in 1962 to measure the capacity of a product to block UV radiation. An SPF of at least 15 is recommended. It takes about 20 minutes without sunscreen for your skin to turn red. A product that is SPF 15 should delay burning by a factor of 15, or about 5 hours or so. Higher SPF ratings give more protection, and are beneficial to those with fair skin.

Besides the sun, injuries will most likely be related to cooking and managing campfires. Using hand protection will prevent many of these burns, as will careful supervision of children near any cooking area.

Burns are traditionally assessed by degree of damage, as described below.

First-Degree Burns

These burns will be very common, such as simple sunburn. The injury will appear red, warm and dry, and will be painful to the touch. These burns frequently affect large areas of the torso; immersion in a cool bath or running cool water over the injury is helpful.

Placing a cool moist cloth on the area will give some relief, as will common anti-inflammatory medicines such as ibuprofen. Aloe vera or zinc-oxide cream is also an effective treatment.

Usually, the discomfort improves after 24 hours or so, as only the superficial skin layer, the epidermis, is affected. Avoid tight clothing and try to wear light fabrics, such as cotton.

Second-Degree Burns

These burns are deeper, going partially through the skin, and will be seen to be moist and have blisters with reddened bases. The area will have a tendency to weep clear or whitish fluid. The area will become somewhat swollen, so remove rings and bracelets.

Treat second-degree burns as follows:

- Run cool water over the injury for 10–15 minutes (avoid ice).
- Give oral pain relief, such as ibuprofen.

- Apply anesthetic ointments or gels.
- Use silver sulfadiazine (Silvadene) creams to help prevent infection.
- Lance only large blisters.
- Avoid peeling off burned skin.
- Apply nonstick skin dressings.

Third-Degree Burns

Third-degree burns involve the full thickness of skin and possibly deeper structures, such as subcutaneous fat and muscle. The burned skin may appear charred or white. The burn may appear indented if significant tissue has been lost.

Third-degree burns will cause dehydration, so giving fluids is essential to keep the patient stable. Cool the burn area with water for 20 minutes, but never immerse in a bath. Celox combat gauze, when wet, forms a gel-like dressing that may provide a helpful barrier. Silver sulfadiazine (Silvadene) cream is helpful in preventing infections in third-degree burns.

Any burn this severe that is larger than, say, 1 inch or so in diameter, usually requires a skin graft to heal completely. A person with third-degree burns over more than 10 percent of the body surface could go into shock, and is in a life-threatening situation.

Natural Burn Remedies

A successful medic will ensure that everyone will have some knowledge regarding alternate burn treatments. Although of limited use for severe burns, many first- and second-degree burns will respond to their effects. There are many different options:

- **Aloe vera.** Studies have shown that aloe vera helps new skin cells form and speeds healing. If you have an aloe plant, cut off a leaf, open it up, and either scoop out the gel or rub the open leaf directly on the burned area 4–6 times daily.
- **Vinegar.** Vinegar works as an astringent and antiseptic and helps to prevent infections. The best way to use vinegar on smaller-sized burns is to make a compress with ½ vinegar and ½ cool water and cover the burn until the compress feels warm, then re-soak the compress and reapply. Alternatively, add vinegar to a cool bath.

- **Witch hazel.** Another "cooling off" treatment for burns is a witch-hazel compress. Use the extract of the bark, which decreases inflammation and soothes a first-degree burn. Soak a compress in full-strength witch hazel and apply to the burned area.
- **Black tea.** The leaves have tannic acid that helps draw heat from a burn. Put 2–3 tea bags in cool water for a few minutes and use the water with compresses or dab on with cotton balls.
- **Baking soda.** Add ¼ cup baking soda to a warm bath and soak for at least 15 minutes or longer if needed, until the water cools off.
- **Raw honey.** Honey has an acidic pH that is inhospitable to bacteria. Apply a generous amount of honey in a thick layer all over the burned area. Cover the honey with cling plastic wrap or waterproof dressings. Use tape to hold the dressing in place. Change the dressing and add more honey at least 3 times a day.

It is important to know that butter or lard, commonly used for burns in the past, will hold in the heat and are not to be used in the treatment of your patient.

Treating burns without a medical system available will require constant care and close observation. Severe fluid losses lead to dangerous consequences for these patients, so always be certain that you do everything possible to keep them well-hydrated. The damage to the skin caused by burns leaves those injured at the mercy of many pathogens, so watch for fevers or other signs of infection.

ANIMAL BITES

In the United States, millions of people are bitten by animals every year. Most animal bites will be puncture wounds on the hands (in adults) and the face, head, and neck (in children). These bites will be relatively small but have the potential to cause dangerous infections.

Most people have, at some time of their life, run afoul of an ornery dog or cat. Domestic pets, including cats, dogs, and small rodents, are the culprits in the grand majority of bite cases. Any of these can lead to infection if ignored, but cat bites inject bacteria into deeper tissue and seem to become contaminated more often.

Besides the trauma associated with the actual bite, various animals carry diseases that can be transmitted to humans. It is possible, for example, to develop tetanus from any animal bite.

Whenever a person has been bitten, the first and most important action is to put on gloves and clean the wound thoroughly with soap and water. Flushing the wound with an irrigation syringe will help remove dirt and bacteria-containing saliva. Be sure to control any bleeding with direct pressure.

Any animal bite should be considered a "dirty" wound and should not be taped, sutured, or stapled shut. If the bite is on the hand, any rings or bracelets should be taken off; if swelling occurs, they may be very difficult to remove later.

Frequent cleansing is the best treatment for a bite wound. Also apply antibiotic ointment to the area, and be sure to watch for signs of infection. You may see redness, swelling, or oozing. In many instances, the site might feel unusually warm to the touch.

Oral antibiotics may be appropriate treatment (especially after a cat bite): Clindamycin (veterinary equivalent: Fish Cin), 300 mg orally every 6 hours, and ciprofloxacin (veterinary equivalent: Fish Flox), 500 mg every 12 hours, in combination would be a good choice, but azithromycin and ampicillin-sulbactam are also options. A tetanus shot is indicated in those who haven't been vaccinated in the last 5 years.

Rabies is a dangerous but, luckily, uncommon disease that can be transmitted by an animal bite. Commonly associated with dogs, wildlife accounts for the grand majority of cases in the United States. Raccoons, opossums, skunks, coyotes, and bats are possible vectors. It is estimated that 40,000 people in the United States receive rabies prevention treatment every year.

A person with rabies is usually symptom-free for a time, which varies in each case. (The average is 30 days or so.) The patient then begins to complain of fatigue, fever, headache, loss of appetite, and fatigue. The site of the bite wound may be itchy or numb. A few days later, evidence of nerve damage appears in the form of irritability, disorientation, hallucination, seizures, and eventually, paralysis. The victim may go into a coma or suffer cardiac or respiratory arrest. Once a person develops the disease, it is usually fatal.

It is important to remember that humans are animals, and you might see bites from this source as well. Approximately 10–15 percent of human bites become infected, because saliva carries 100 million bacteria per milliliter.

Although it would be extraordinarily rare to get rabies as a result of a human bite, transmission of hepatitis, tetanus, herpes, syphilis, and even HIV is possible. Treat as you would any contaminated wound.

SNAKE BITES

In a grid-down scenario, you will likely find yourself out in the woods a lot more frequently, gathering firewood, hunting, and foraging for edible wild plants. As such, you may encounter a snake or two. Most snakes aren't venomous, but even non-venomous snakebites may cause infections.

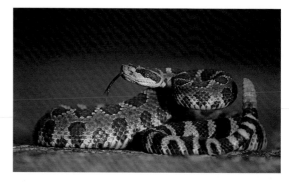

Venom differs from poison. While poisons are absorbed by the skin or digestive system, venoms must enter the tissues or blood directly. Therefore, it is usually not dangerous to drink snake venom unless you have, say, a cut in your mouth. (Don't try it, though.)

North America has two kinds of venomous snakes: pit vipers (rattlesnakes, water moccasins) and elapids (coral snakes). One or more of these snakes can be found almost everywhere in the continental United States. A member of another viper family, the common adder, is the only venomous snake in the United Kingdom, but it and other adders are common throughout Europe, except for Ireland.

These snakes generally have hollow fangs through which they deliver venom. Snakes are most active during the warmer months, and therefore most bite injuries are seen then. Not every bite from a venomous snake transfers its venom to the victim: 25–30 percent of these bites will show no ill effects. This probably has to do with the duration of time the snake has its fangs in its victim.

To prevent snakebite, wear good, solid, high-top boots and long pants when hiking in the wilderness. Treading heavily creates ground vibrations and noise, which will often cause snakes to move away. Snakes have no outer ear, so they "hear" ground vibrations better than those in the air caused by shouting.

Many snakes are active at night, especially in warm weather. Some activities of daily survival, such as gathering firewood, are inadvisable without a good light source. In the wilderness, it's important to look where you're putting your hands and feet. Be especially careful around areas where snakes might like to hide, such as in or under hollow logs, under rocks, or in old shelters. Wearing heavy gloves would be a reasonable precaution.

A snake doesn't always slither away after it bites you. It's likely that it still has more venom that it can inject, so move out of its territory or abolish the threat in any way you can. Killing the snake, however, may not render it harmless: The severed head can reflexively bite for a period of time.

Snake bites that cause a burning pain immediately are likely to have venom in them. Swelling at the site may begin as soon as 5 minutes afterwards, and may travel up the affected area. Pit-viper bites tend to cause bruising and blisters at the site of the wound. Numbness may be noted in the area bitten, or perhaps on the lips or face. Some victims describe a metallic or other strange taste in their mouths.

With pit vipers, bruising is not uncommon and a serious bite might start to cause spontaneous bleeding from the nose or gums. Coral snake bites, however, will cause mental and nerve issues, such as twitching, confusion, and slurred speech. Later, nerve damage may cause difficulty with swallowing and breathing, followed by total paralysis.

Coral snakes appear very similar to their look-alike, the nonvenomous king snake. They both have red, yellow, and black bands and are commonly confused with each other. As the old saying goes, "red touches yellow, kill a fellow; red touches black, venom it lacks." This adage only applies to coral snakes in North America, however.

Coral snakes are not as aggressive as pit vipers and will prefer fleeing to attacking. Once they bite you, however, they tend to hold on; pit vipers prefer to bite and let go quickly. Unlike coral snakes, pit vipers may not relinquish their territory to you, so prepare to possibly be bitten again.

The treatment for a venomous snake bite is antivenin, an animal or human serum with antibodies capable of neutralizing a specific biological toxin. This product will probably be unavailable in a long-term survival situation. The following strategy, therefore, will be useful:

1. Keep the victim calm. Stress increases blood flow, thereby endangering the patient by speeding the venom into the system.
2. Stop all movement of the injured extremity. Movement will move the venom into the circulation system faster, so do your best to keep the limb still.

3. Clean the wound thoroughly to remove any venom that isn't deep in the wound.
4. Remove rings and bracelets from an affected extremity. Swelling is likely to occur.
5. Position the extremity below the level of the heart; this also slows the transport of venom.
6. Wrap with compression bandages as you would an orthopedic injury, but continue it further up the limb than usual. Bandaging should begin 2–4 inches above the bite (towards the heart), winding around and moving up, then back down over the bite and past it towards the hand or foot.
7. Keep the wrapping about as tight as when dressing a sprained ankle. If it is too tight, the patient will reflexively move the limb, and move the venom around. Do not use tourniquets, which will do more harm than good.
8. Draw a circle, if possible, around the affected area. As time progresses, you will see improvement or worsening at the site more clearly. This is a useful strategy to follow any local reaction or infection.

The limb should then be rested, and perhaps immobilized with a splint or sling. Keep the patient on bed rest, with the bite site lower than the heart for 24–48 hours. This strategy also works for bites from venomous lizards, such as Gila monsters.

Medical experts do not recommend making an incision and trying to suck out the venom with your mouth. If done more than 3 minutes after the actual bite, it would remove perhaps 1/1,000 of the venom and could cause damage or infection to the bitten area. A Sawyer Extractor™ (a syringe with a suction cup) is more modern, but is also fairly ineffective in eliminating more than a small amount of the venom. These methods usually fail because of the speed at which the venom is absorbed.

Snake bites cause fewer infections than bites from, say, cats, dogs, or humans. As such, antibiotics are used less often in these cases.

INVERTEBRATE BITES AND STINGS

In a survival scenario, you will see a million invertebrates, such as insects and spiders, for every snake; so many, indeed, that you can expect to regularly get bitten by them. Insect bites usually cause pain, local redness, itching, and swelling, but are rarely life threatening. The hairs and fibers on

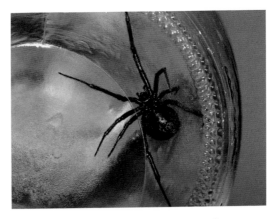

Southern Black Widow Spider

some caterpillars carry toxins that can also deliver a painful sting that, unless the victim has a severe allergic reaction, is not life threatening.

The invertebrates to watch out for are arachnids—black widow spiders, brown recluse spiders, and scorpions. Many of these bites can inject toxins that could cause serious damage. Of course, we are talking about the bite itself, not disease that may be passed on by the insect. This topic is discussed in the section on mosquito-borne illness.

Bee and Wasp Stings

For most sting victims, the offender will be a bee, wasp, or hornet (a type of wasp). A bee will leave its stinger in the victim, but wasps take their stingers with them and can sting again. Even though you won't get stung again by the same bee, they send out a scent that informs nearby bees that an attack is under way. As such, you should leave the area, whether the culprit was a bee or wasp.

The best way to reduce any reaction to bee venom is to remove the bee stinger as quickly as possible. Pull it out with tweezers or, if possible, scrape it out with your fingernail. The longer bee stingers are allowed to remain in the body, the higher the chance for a severe reaction.

Most bee and wasp stings heal with little or no treatment. For those that experience only local reactions, the following actions will be sufficient:

1. Clean the area thoroughly.
2. Remove the stinger, if visible, with tweezers.
3. Place cold packs and anesthetic ointments to relieve discomfort and local swelling.
4. Control itching and redness with oral antihistamines, such as Benadryl or Claritin.
5. Give acetaminophen or ibuprofen to reduce discomfort.
6. Apply antibiotic ointments to prevent infection.

Application of topical essential oils (after removing the stinger) can also help. Use *Helichrysum* (a genus of sunflower), tea tree, or peppermint oil, applying 1–2 drops to the affected area 3 times a day. A baking soda paste (baking soda mixed with a small amount of water) may be useful when applied to a sting wound.

Although most of these injuries are relatively minor, quite a few people are allergic to the toxins in the stings. Some are so allergic that they will have an anaphylactic reaction. Instead of just local symptoms, such as rashes and itching, they will experience dizziness, difficulty breathing, faintness, or all of these. Severe swelling is seen in some, which can be life threatening if it closes the person's airways.

Spider Bites

Although large spiders, such as tarantulas, cause painful bites, most spider bites don't even break the skin. In temperate climates, two spiders are to be especially feared: the black widow and the brown recluse.

The black widow spider is about ½ inch long and is active mostly at night. They rarely invade your home, but can be found in outbuildings like barns and garages. The female southern black widow (*Latrodectus mactans*) has a red hourglass pattern on the underside of its abdomens; males and juveniles vary in color and may not have the hourglass, and some widow species also vary from the southern black widow in appearance. Although the black widow's bite has very potent venom that can damage the nervous system, the effects on each individual victim vary considerably.

A black widow bite will appear red and raised, and two small puncture marks may be visible at the site of the wound. Severe pain at the site is usually the first symptom and appears soon after the bite. Following this, may appear:

- Muscle cramps
- Abdominal pain
- Weakness
- Shakiness
- Nausea and vomiting
- Fainting
- Chest pain
- Difficulty breathing
- Disorientation

Each person will present with a variable combination and degree of the symptoms listed above. The very young and the elderly are more seriously affected than most. In your exam, you can expect rises in both heart rate and blood pressure.

The brown recluse spider is, well, brown, and has legs about 1 inch long. Unlike most spiders, it only has six eyes instead of eight, but they are so small it is difficult to identify the species from this characteristic.

Victims of brown recluse bites report them to be painless at first, but then may experience the following symptoms:

- Itching
- Pain, sometimes severe, after several hours
- Fever
- Nausea and vomiting
- Blisters

The venom of the brown recluse is thought to be more potent than a rattlesnake's, although much less is injected in its bite. Substances in the venom disrupt soft tissue, which leads to local breakdown of blood vessels, skin, and fat. This process, seen in severe cases, leads to necrosis (death of tissue) immediately surrounding the bite. Areas affected may be extensive.

Once bitten, the human body activates its immune response as a result, and can go haywire, destroying red blood cells and kidney tissue, and hampering the ability of blood to clot appropriately. These effects can lead to coma and eventually death. Almost all deaths from brown recluse bites are recorded in children.

The treatment for spider bites includes the following:

- Thorough washing of the bite area
- Ice, applied to painful and swollen areas
- Pain medications, such as acetaminophen (Tylenol)
- Enforced bed rest
- Warm baths for those with muscle cramps (black widow bites only; do not apply heat to the area with brown recluse bites)
- Antibiotics, to prevent secondary bacterial infection

Home remedies include making a paste out of baking soda or aspirin and applying it to the wound. The same method, using olive oil and turmeric in combination, is a time-honored tradition. Dried basil has also been suggested; crush it between your fingers until it becomes a fine dust, then apply to the bite. Be aware that these methods may be variable in their effect from patient to patient.

Although antivenins exist and may be lifesaving for venomous spider and scorpion stings, these will be scarce in the aftermath of a major disaster. Luckily, most cases that are not severe will subside over the course of a few days, but the sickest patients will be nearly untreatable without the antivenin.

Scorpion Stings

Most scorpions are harmless; in the United States, only the bark scorpion of the Southwest desert has toxins that can cause severe symptoms. In other areas of the world, however, a scorpion sting may be lethal. Some scorpions may reach several inches long; they have pincers and, as with other arachnids, eight legs. They inject venom through a barb at the end of their tails. They are most commonly active at night.

The nervous system is most often affected from a bark scorpion sting. Symptoms of scorpion stings may include the following:

- Pain, numbness, tingling, or all of these, in the area of the sting
- Sweating
- Weakness
- Increased saliva output

† Restlessness or twitching
† Irritability
† Difficulty swallowing
† Rapid breathing and heart rate

When you have diagnosed a scorpion sting, do the following:

- Wash the area with soap and water.
- Remove jewelry from affected limb (swelling may occur).
- Apply cold compresses to decrease pain.
- Give an antihistamine, such as diphenhydramine (Benadryl).

If you do the following things quickly, this may slow the venom's spread:

- Keep your patient calm to slow down the spread of venom.
- Limit food intake if throat is swollen.
- Give pain relievers, such as ibuprofen or acetaminophen, but avoid narcotics, as they may suppress breathing.
- Don't cut in the wound or use suction to attempt to remove venom.

Although not likely available in an austere environment, there is an anti-venin that eliminates symptoms in children (the group most severely affected) after 4 hours.

HEAD INJURIES

Head injuries can be soft-tissue injuries (brain, scalp, blood vessels) or bony injuries (skull, facial bones). Damage is usually caused by direct impact, such as a laceration in the scalp or a fracture of the cranium, the part of the skull that contains the brain. Anyone with a traumatic injury to the head must always be observed closely, as symptoms may take time to develop.

An "open" head injury means that the skull has been penetrated with possible exposure of the brain tissue. If the skull is not fractured, it is referred to as a "closed" injury. Damage can also be caused by the rebound of the brain against the inside walls of the skull; this may result in rupture of blood vessels and bleeding (a contrecoup injury). There may be no obvious penetrating wound in this case. An example of this would be the violent shaking of an infant.

The brain requires blood and oxygen to function normally. A traumatic brain injury (TBI) that causes bleeding or swelling inside the skull may increase the intracranial pressure. This causes the heart to work harder to get blood and oxygen into the brain. Hematoma (blood accumulation) could occur within the brain tissue or between the layers of tissue covering the brain. Pressure that is high enough could actually cause a portion of the brain to push downward through the base of the skull. Known as a "brain herniation," without modern medical care, this almost invariably leads to death.

Most head injuries result in only a laceration to the scalp and a swelling at the site of impact. Cuts on the scalp or face may bleed heavily, as there are many small blood vessels that travel through this area. This bleeding does not have to signify internal damage; most cases can be treated as any other laceration. There are a number of signs and symptoms, however, that might help in identifying patients who are more seriously affected. They include the following:

- Loss of consciousness
- Convulsions (seizures)
- Worsening headache
- Nausea and vomiting
- Bruising around eyes and ears ("raccoon sign")

- Bleeding or fluid leakage from ears and nose
- Confusion, apathy, or drowsiness
- One pupil more dilated than the other (nerve compression)
- Indentation of the skull

A concussion is a head injury that results in changes in brain function, even for a very short period of time and does not necessarily include loss of consciousness. Indeed, most concussions are not associated with loss of consciousness.

If brief loss of consciousness does occur, the patient will usually awaken somewhat "foggy," and may be unclear as to how the injury occurred or the events shortly before or after. Effects are usually temporary but can include headaches (the most common symptom), ringing in the ears, dizziness, and problems with concentration, memory, balance, and coordination. They may appear sluggish or tired.

It is important to be certain that the patient, once awake, has regained normal motor function. In other words, make sure they can move all their extremities with normal range and strength. Even so, rest is prescribed for a day or two, so that they may be closely watched. Acetaminophen should be given for headache instead of aspirin or ibuprofen, because of the risk of bleeding.

It's OK to let your patient get some sleep. Once asleep, it might be appropriate to awaken them about every 2 hours to make sure that they can be aroused and have developed none of the danger signals mentioned.

In most cases, a concussion causes no permanent damage if further trauma is avoided. Multiple episodes of head trauma over time, however— as in the case of boxers or some other athletes—can lead to long-term brain damage. This can manifest as follows:

- Memory deficits
- Personality changes
- Sleep disturbances
- Seizures
- Psychological problems such as depression
- Disorders of taste and smell
- Sensitivity to light and noise

If the period of unconsciousness is more than 10 minutes in length, you must suspect the possibility of significant injury. Vital signs, such as pulse, respiration rate, and blood pressure, should be monitored closely. The patient's head should be immobilized, in case there is damage to the spine. Verify that the airway is clear, and remove any possible obstructions. Without advanced care, this person will be in a life-threatening situation, with few options, if consciousness is not regained.

SPRAINS AND STRAINS

Bones, joints, muscles, and tendons give the body support and locomotion, and there is no substitute for having all your parts in good working order. The amount of work these structures will be called upon to do after a disaster will be greatly increased. Therefore, the medic will expect to see more injuries; it is important to know how to identify and treat these problems.

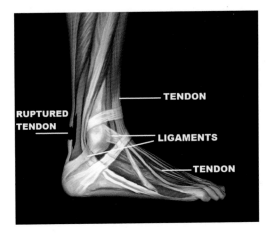

Many people have heard of ligaments, tendons, sprains, and strains but have little idea of what they really are. Therefore, let's define some anatomical terms:

Joint—the physical point of connection between two bones, usually enabling a certain range of motion, for example, the knee or elbow joint

Ligament—the fibrous tissue that connects one bone to another, oftentimes across a joint

Tendon—tissue that extends from muscle to connect to bone

Sprain—an injury where a ligament is excessively stretched by forcing a joint beyond its normal range of motion

Strain—when the muscle or its connection to the bone (tendon) is partially torn as a result of an injury

Rupture—a complete tear through a ligament or muscle

Sprains

Our joints are truly marvels of engineering. They help provide mobility and locomotion and sometimes bear an incredible amount of stress without mishap. They are moving parts, however, and moving parts wear down. In a disaster, our level of physical exertion may increase; the risk of injury to the joints increases as well.

You can expect the most common sprains in your group to involve the ankle, wrist, knee, or finger. The most likely signs and symptoms are bruising, swelling, and pain.

Treatment for most sprains is relatively straightforward and follows the easy-to-remember RICES protocol:

Rest. It is important to avoid further injury by not testing the injured joint. Stop whatever actions led to the injury, and you will have the best chance to recover fully.

Ice. Cold therapy decreases both swelling and pain. The earlier it is applied, the more likely it will speed up the healing process. If you're in the wilderness, have some instant cold packs in your backpack, as ice may be unavailable.

Cold therapy should be performed several times a day for 20–30 minutes or so each time for the first 24–48 hours. This is followed each time by applying compression.

Compression. A compression bandage is useful to decrease swelling and should be applied after each cold therapy. This will also help provide support to the joint. After applying some padding to the area, securely wrap an elastic bandage, starting below the joint and working your way up beyond it.

Any tingling, increased pain, or numbness tells you that the wrap is too tight and should be loosened. An excessively tight wrap may affect the circulation and cause fingertips to turn white or even blue.

Elevation. Elevate the sprain above the level of the heart. This will help decrease swelling at the site of the injury. By elevating the leg, you allow inflammatory fluid to process itself back into your circulation and aid the healing process, or at least not impede it.

This also works for swollen ankles due to chronic medical problems, like high blood pressure; even pregnant women achieve relief from swollen ankles in this fashion.

Stabilization. Immobilizing the injury will prevent further damage. This may be accomplished by the compression bandage alone or may require a splint or a cast. If the patient is unable to place much weight on the joint, this strategy will be especially useful.

Splints may be commercially produced, such as the very useful SAM (structural aluminum malleable) splint, or may be improvised with sticks and cloth or pillows and duct tape. Make sure the injured joint is immobile after placement of the splint.

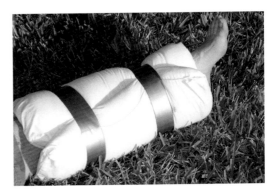

Pillow splint

How can you tell the difference between a sprain and a fracture? Sometimes it's quite easy, as when a straight bone is suddenly "zig-zag" in shape. Often it's quite difficult to determine without modern diagnostic tests.

You can, however, look for one or more of these signs that an injury may relate to a fracture rather than a sprain:

- A fracture will generally have more pronounced swelling and bruising.
- A fracture is generally so painful that no traction or pressure may be placed on the injury.
- A fracture may have a deep cut in the area of the injury (called an "open" fracture, which is particularly dangerous because of the risk of infection).
- A fracture may show motion in an area beyond the joint (if your finger suddenly has five knuckles, you probably broke it).
- A fracture may present a grating sensation when the point of the break is pressed.

For sprains, ibuprofen serves as both an anti-inflammatory and pain reliever. Most sprains heal well over time using the RICES protocol, pain relievers, and a lot of rest. Others, however, such as severe knee sprains with torn or ruptured ligaments, may heal completely only with the aid of surgical intervention.

It's important to get joint issues dealt with while we still have modern medicine to help us. If you need surgery to fix a bad knee, do it now. In uncertain times, you (and your joints) want to be in the best shape possible to face the challenges ahead.

Strains

By far, the most frequently seen strain will be to the back muscles. Strains, especially back strains, involve injury to the muscle and their tendons (which connects them to the bone). As the lower part of the back holds the majority of the body's weight, you can expect the most trouble here. Some of these injuries are preventable with some simple precautions:

- Every morning you should perform some stretching, to increase blood flow to cold, stiff muscles and joints.
- When you lift a heavy object, such as a backpack, keep your back straight and let your legs perform the work.
- The object should be close to your body as you lift it. (Don't reach for it.)
- For packs, keep the weight on the hips rather than the shoulders.
- If you are on rocky or unstable terrain, consider using a walking stick for balance. Remember, any weight-lifting action that you perform while being off-balance is likely to result in a strained muscle.

Moist heat therapy seems to be effective for relief in back strains. Ibuprofen is an excellent anti-inflammatory and pain reliever for these types of injury. For muscle injuries, prescription relaxants such as diazepam (Valium) or cyclobenzaprine (Flexeril™) will also provide relief. If these are not available, the patient will benefit from mild massage.

Common herbal pain relievers for orthopedic injuries include direct application of oil—including wintergreen, *Helichrysum*, peppermint, clove, or diluted arnica—to the affected area. Blends of these oils may also be used. Herbal teas that may give relief are valerian root, willow underbark, ginger, passionflower, feverfew, and turmeric. Mix warm tea with raw honey several times a day.

Some sprains and strains heal well over time with the therapy described above. Other injuries may cause chronic pain and eventual degeneration of the joint. It will be difficult to foretell the progress of an injured joint without modern diagnostic imaging.

DISLOCATIONS

A dislocation is an injury in which a bone is pulled out of its joint by some type of trauma. Dislocations commonly occur in shoulders, fingers, and elbows, but knees, ankles, and hips may also be affected. The joint involved looks visibly abnormal and is unusable. Bruising, pain, numbness, or all of these often accompany the injury.

CROOKED AND SWOLLEN

DISLOCATED FINGER

A subluxation occurs when a dislocation is momentary and the bone slips back into its joint spontaneously. Subluxations can be treated the same way that sprains are, using the RICES method. It should be noted that the traditional medical definition of subluxation is somewhat different from the chiropractic one.

Of course, if there is medical care readily available, the patient should go directly to the local emergency room. General anesthesia if often used to resolve the problem. Off the grid, however, you will probably have to correct the dislocation yourself. This is known as performing a "reduction" of the injury.

Reduction is best performed very soon after the dislocation, before significant swelling occurs. Not only does reducing the dislocation decrease the pain experienced by the victim, but, if performed correctly, will lessen the damage to all the blood vessels and nerves that run along the injury.

Expect significant pain on the part of the patient during the actual procedure, however. Some pain relievers, such as ibuprofen, may be useful to decrease discomfort from the reduction. Prescription muscle relaxers, such as cyclobenzaprine (Flexeril), are also helpful.

The use of traction will greatly aid your attempt to fix the problem. Traction is the act of pulling the dislocated bone away from the joint to give the bone room to slip back into place.

The procedure is as follows:

1. Stabilize the joint from which the bone was dislocated (the shoulder, for example).
2. Using a firm but slow pulling action, pull the bone away from the joint. This will make space for the bone to realign.
3. Use your other hand (or preferably a helper's hands) to push the dislocated portion of the bone so that it will be in line again with the joint socket. The bone will naturally want to revert to its normal position in the joint.
4. After the reduction is complete and judged successful, immobilize the joint to prevent further injury (see next section).

Some dislocations, such as that of a finger, may take as little as 2–3 weeks to regain normal function. Others, such as hip dislocations, may take many months to heal.

FRACTURES

If enough force is applied, an injury to soft tissue can damage the skeletal structure underneath. When a bone is broken, it is termed a "fracture." There are several types of fractures, but for our purposes let's assume that they are either "open" or "closed." A closed fracture is when there is a break in the bone, but the skin is intact. In open fractures, the skin is pierced by the broken bone or there is some other penetrating trauma. The end of the bone may be above or below the level of the skin.

Needless to say, there is usually more blood loss and infection associated with an open wound. The infection may be deep in the skin (cellulitis), the blood (septicemia), or the bone itself (osteomyelitis) and could be life threatening if not treated. If poorly managed, a closed fracture can become an open fracture.

The diagnosis of a broken bone can be simple, as when the bone is obviously deformed, or difficult, as in a minimal, "hairline" fracture. X-rays can be helpful to differentiate a small fracture from a severe sprain, but that technology won't be available in a power-down situation.

Dealing with a fractured bone involves first evaluating the injured area. Use EMT scissors to cut away the clothing over the injury. This will prevent further injury that may occur if the patient is made to remove their own clothing. Check the site for bleeding and the presence of an open wound; if present, stop the bleeding before proceeding further.

Fractures may cause damage to the patient's circulation in the limb affected, so it is important to check the area beyond the level of the injury for changes in coloration (white or blue instead of normal skin color) and for strong and steady pulses. Usually, normal color returns to skin in the fingertips within 2 seconds of applying pressure and then releasing (capillary refill time.

To find out what a strong pulse feels like, place two fingers on the side of your neck until you feel your neck arteries pulsing. You will do this same action on, say, the wrist, if the patient has broken his or her arm. Lightly prick the patient in the same area with a toothpick to make sure they have normal sensation. If not, the nerve has been injured.

If the bone has not deformed the extremity, a simple splint will immobilize the fracture, prevent further injury to soft tissues, and promote appropriate healing. Often, however, the bone will be obviously bent or otherwise deformed, and the fracture must be reduced, as we discussed with dislocations. Although this will be painful, normal healing and complete recovery will not occur until the two ends of the broken bone are realigned to their original position.

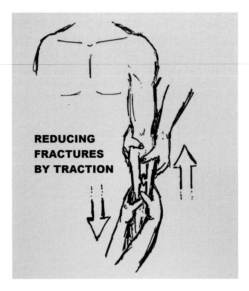

REDUCING
FRACTURES
BY TRACTION

Splint the extremity in place immediately after performing the reduction. Traction to keep the bone straight may be necessary in many cases. In an open fracture, thorough washing of the wound is absolutely necessary to prevent internal infection. Infection will invariably occur in a dirty wound, even if the reduction is successful. Therefore, antibiotics are important to prevent complications, such as osteomyelitis. Always check the pulses and capillary refill time after the reduction is performed; this will ensure adequate circulation beyond the level of the injury.

It is very important to immobilize the fractured bone in such a fashion that it is allowed to heal. When you are responsible for the complete healing of the broken bone, remember that the splint should immobilize it in a position that it normally would assume in routine function.

Splints can be commercially produced or may be improvised, using straight sticks and bandannas or T-shirts to immobilize the area. Another option is to fold a pillow around the injury and duct tape it in place.

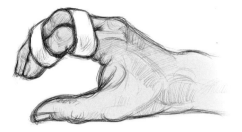

FRACTURED FINGER BUDDY

Fractured fingers and toes may be splinted by taping them to an adjoining digit, called the "buddy method." There are small manufactured splints that will also do the job. Neck injuries may be particularly serious, and an investment should be made in purchasing a good neck collar.

For most fractures, you will want to consider the placement of a cast to enforce immobilization. Casting material using plaster of Paris or fiberglass is easy to obtain and lasts a long time. It's a useful addition to any medical storage.

When placing a cast, you will first start with a liner of cotton known as a "stockinette." Then, you will need rolls of padding to form a barrier between the skin and the cast. Rolls of plaster of Paris or fiberglass are then immersed in water for 20 seconds or so. Wring out the excess water. (Keep the end of the roll between your fingers or it will stick and be difficult to find.)

Then, begin to slowly roll the casting material around the area of the fracture, smoothing it out as you go along. Advance one-half of the thickness of the roll as you go from beyond the fracture towards the torso. You will want perhaps three layers of casting material on the area, more in places where there is a bony prominence, such as the wrist.

Each fracture is casted somewhat differently, and stockinettes, padding, and casting rolls are available in different widths and lengths appropriate to the particular fracture. Although oscillating saws are used today to remove casts, special heavy-duty shears are still available for the purpose, although some effort is required to use them.

Your goal is to immobilize the fracture in a position of function. Use padding under the splint or cast to keep the injured area stable and protected. Most fractures require 6–8 weeks to form a callous, newly formed tissue that will reunite the broken ends of the bone. Larger bones or more complicated injuries take longer to "knit" together. If the fracture is not realigned well, the function of the affected extremity can be permanently compromised.

Rib Fractures and Pneumothorax

Rib fractures are commonly treated by firmly taping the affected area, as it is the motion of breathing that causes the pain associated with the injury. Although reduction is usually not necessary, taping the area may help provide pain relief.

Rib fractures become more serious if the fracture punctures a lung. This causes a pneumothorax (collapsed lung), a condition in which air from the puncture enters the chest cavity, compressing the lung and collapsing the organ.

Although a person with a rib fracture will complain of pain with breathing, a person with a pneumothorax will have signs of bluish skin coloration (cyanosis), distended neck veins, and signs of shock. If you use a stethoscope, you will hear the sounds *snap, crackle, and pop*, familiarly associated with Rice Krispies™ cereal when you listen to the lungs, or perhaps no breath sounds at all from the affected area.

If the pneumothorax has become life threatening, known as a "tension pneumothorax," you may have to decompress the lung. This should only be attempted if it's clear the patient will die without this action being taken.

Clean the area of the chest above the third rib, midway between the top of the shoulder and the nipple. Using a sharp object no wider than a pencil, poke a hole *above* the rib (the blood vessels travel below the rib) deep enough to hear air pass through. A large-gauge (14 or larger) decompression needle is commercially available.

Your goal is to provide a way for the air to continue to escape from the incision you made but not to go back in. This is called a "chest seal" and manufactured versions are available. To improvise, take a square of plastic wrap or a plastic bag and firmly tape it above the skin incision on three sides only. This will serve as a valve, which allows air to escape from the chest cavity and the lung to reinflate.

Inflammatory or bloody fluid is likely to accumulate in many lung wounds. You will have to rig a drainage system to keep fluid from preventing adequate air passage. A rubber tube connected to a jar placed below the patient may perform this duty by using gravity. It will not, however, be as efficient as the electric suction systems available at your local hospital. It's important to realize that chest wounds will be difficult to recover from without advanced care.

AMPUTATION

In rare circumstances, damage to a limb may be so extensive that it cannot be saved. Amputation is the surgical removal of all or part of an extremity. This procedure is performed on arms, legs, hands, feet, fingers, or toes. The closer to the torso that the amputation was performed, the higher the death rate will be.

Amputation, even in a survival situation, is a last resort. In many cases, your patient will not survive it. At least 25 percent of American Civil War soldiers undergoing the procedure by trained personnel lost their lives because of bleeding or infection.

Having said that, there are various reasons why amputation might be necessary:

- Damaged blood vessels that fail to provide oxygen to tissue
- Extensive injury from trauma or burns
- Cancerous tumors
- Severe frostbite
- Gangrene

Look for the following to identify where to cut and how much to remove:

- Where an extremity loses a pulse
- Areas when a limb loses normal temperature
- Areas of reddened skin (infection) or blackened skin (gangrene)
- The place where the extremity is no longer sensitive to touch
- Areas where the bone has been crushed beyond repair

The following are basic measures to increase the chances of a successful amputation:

- Sedate the patient as much as possible.
- Clean the damaged area with Betadine or other antiseptics before the procedure.
- Use sterile gloves in a sterile field.
- Remove debris and bits of shattered bone.
- Tie off bleeding blood vessels.
- Preserve an adequate amount of living tissue to cover the exposed end of the bone.

- Shorten and smooth the bone enough to decrease irritation to the covering soft tissue.
- Stitch remaining muscle to the bone lining (periosteum), which is difficult without special equipment.
- Before closing completely, place a drain (discussed earlier in this book) to enable blood and inflammatory fluid to leave the surgical site.
- Adequately close the wound with sutures or staples.
- Change dressings regularly.
- Observe for infection and, if present, start a course of antibiotics.

Amputation is a procedure we hope you will never have to consider. In severe injuries, however, it may be an avenue of last resort.

VII.

✚ ✚ ✚

CHRONIC MEDICAL PROBLEMS

As a caregiver in a long-term survival scenario, you cannot expect that everyone under your care will start off in perfect health. It is likely that one or more members of your family or group will have a long-standing medical issue that cannot be ignored. Thyroid malfunction, diabetes, and heart disease are just some of these issues. They require medications that will not be manufactured in times of trouble. You must, therefore, think "outside the box" to formulate a medical strategy for these patients that does not include modern technology.

It goes without saying that medical conditions that are poorly controlled now could be completely out of control in a survival setting. The most important way to preserve your family's health will be to have any chronic conditions appropriately treated and monitored *before* a catastrophe.

In this section we discuss some chronic problems with which the medic may have to deal. If you ever find yourself on your own, having a plan in place will increase your effectiveness as caregiver and improve the health of the community.

THYROID DISEASE

The thyroid gland is positioned just in front of and below the Adam's apple (laryngeal prominence) and produces hormones that help regulate your metabolism. The organ produces substances that regulate growth, energy, and the body's use of other hormones and vitamins. Thyroid conditions usually involve the production of either too little or too much of these hormones. These malfunctions are more commonly seen in women.

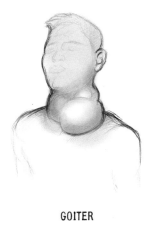

GOITER

A thyroid problem that might be common in an austere setting is the development of a goiter, a lump on the thyroid. This is the result of a deficiency of iodine in the body and is one of the reasons why iodine is added to common table salt, making it "iodized." Potassium iodide tablets may be a treatment option if no other source of iodine is available. It should be noted that iodine-containing drugs should not be administered to those with allergies to seafood.

Hyperthyroidism

Hyperthyroidism is the excessive production of thyroid hormone. Determination of thyroid malfunction depends on certain blood tests and sometimes a scan of the gland. These modalities will be gone in a collapse, so it's important to learn what a person with elevated thyroid levels looks like. The following are some common signs and symptoms of this condition in adults:

- Insomnia
- Hand tremors
- Nervousness
- Feeling excessively hot in normal or cold temperatures
- Eyes appearing to be bulging out or "staring"
- Frequent bowel movements
- Losing weight despite normal or increased appetite

- Excessive sweating
- Weight loss
- Menstrual irregularities
- Growth and puberty issues (children)
- Muscle weakness, chest pain, and shortness of breath (elderly)

Poorly controlled hyperthyroidism can lead to a condition known as "thyroid storm," in which large levels of hormone have major effects on the heart and brain. All the above symptoms may combine with elevated heart rate and blood pressure to endanger the patient's life.

Treatment of hyperthyroidism involves medications such as propylthiouracil and methimazole, which block thyroid function. These medications should be stockpiled if you're aware of a member of your group with hyperthyroidism, as the drugs will be hard to find if modern medical care is no longer available. Iodide is also useful in blocking the excessive production of thyroid hormone, and can be found in kelp in good quantity. Unfortunately, the use of iodides, while a known treatment, may actually worsen the condition in some cases.

Dietary restriction of nicotine, caffeine, alcohol and other substances that alter metabolism will be useful as well. Vitamins C and B12 are thought to have a beneficial effect on those with this condition. L-carnitine is also beneficial in that it may lower thyroid hormone levels without damaging the gland.

Foods that are thought to depress production of thyroid hormone include cabbage, cauliflower, broccoli, Brussels sprout, and spinach. In addition, foods high in antioxidants are thought to reduce free radicals that might be involved in hyperthyroidism. These include blueberries, cherries, tomatoes, squash, and bell peppers, among many others.

Hypothyroidism

More commonly seen than hyperthyroidism, hypothyroidism is the failure to produce *enough* thyroid hormone. Various causes of low thyroid levels exist, such as certain drugs or exposure to radiation. Also, the immune system sometimes misfires and targets the thyroid. The following are the most commonly seen signs and symptoms of hypothyroidism in adults:

- Fatigue
- Intolerance to cold

- ♆ Constipation
- ♆ Poor appetite
- ♆ Weight gain
- ♆ Dry skin
- ♆ Hair loss
- ♆ Hoarseness
- ♆ Depression
- ♆ Menstrual irregularity
- ♆ Poor growth (in children)

Long-standing untreated hypothyroidism may result in thickened skin, hair loss (alopecia), vocal changes, and swelling. Hypothyroidism in a pregnant woman may cause birth defects in the baby.

The treatment of this condition is based on the oral replacement of the missing hormone, thyroxine. Such replacements come in a variety of dosages, and it is important to determine the appropriate one for your patient while modern medical care is still available. The lowest dose that will maintain normal thyroid levels is indicated to avoid hyperthyroidism.

Besides standard thyroid medications, such as Synthroid™ and Levothroid™, there are a number of other remedies that may improve hypothyroidism. A number of thyroid extracts are available that consist of desiccated and powdered pig or cow thyroid gland. The effects of these extracts may be variable. Having said this, in the absence of modern medications, it is better than nothing.

From a dietary standpoint, you should avoid foods that depress thyroid functions, including the following:

- Cauliflower
- Broccoli
- Brussels sprout
- Spinach
- Cabbage

A number of natural supplements, such as Thyromine, are commercially available. They are combinations of various herbs that are touted as beneficial for both low and high thyroid conditions. Your experience may vary.

DIABETES

Diabetes is a common, yet devastating, disease characterized by high sugar (glucose) levels in the blood. Uncontrolled diabetes is known to cause damage to various organs, such as the kidneys, eyes, and heart. The incidence of the disease has been increasing over time in developed countries, perhaps because of issues relating to obesity.

Diabetes is especially problematic for the survival medic in that the medications used to treat the worst cases are unlikely to be produced in a grid-down scenario. Diabetic medications, such as insulin, lose potency over time. Therefore, an alternative strategy to keep diabetics from losing complete control of their blood sugar will have to be formulated.

There are two types of diabetes. Type 1 results from the failure of the pancreas to produce insulin. Insulin is a hormone that controls the level of sugar in your system. The destruction of the cells in the pancreas that produce insulin is thought to be caused by an autoimmune response. This means that the body's own immune system attacks parts of itself. Type 1 diabetes is often first diagnosed in childhood.

Type 2 diabetes is more commonly the result of the resistance of the cells in your body to the insulin produced by the pancreas. Obesity is thought to be a major factor. In type 2 diabetes, certain cells do not respond appropriately to insulin. Glucose fails to enter these cells and, therefore, it accumulates in the blood. High blood sugar is known as "hyperglycemia."

Diabetes (mild or severe) may also develop in some pregnancies, even in nondiabetic women. Some believe that those who get diabetes during their pregnancies may be prone to diabetic issues later in life.

There are three classic symptoms of diabetes:

- Extreme thirst
- Excessive hunger
- Frequent urination

Uncontrolled diabetes causes eye and kidney problems, leading to blindness and renal failure. It worsens coronary artery disease, increasing the chances for heart attacks and other cardiac issues. Weight loss may occur despite the consumption of more food; the cells cannot access the glucose in the blood for energy to produce mass.

In a person with diabetes, cuts and scrapes, especially in the extremities, are slow to heal. Over time, nerve damage occurs, which causes numbness, pins-and-needles sensations, and much worse. Many severely uncontrolled diabetics may require amputation.

Type 2 diabetes is most often seen in older, heavier, and less active individuals. Weight control and close attention to controlling the amounts of carbohydrates (which the body turns into sugars) in the diet is important. In some cases, decreasing excess weight and eating frequent small meals may reverse type 2 diabetes in its entirety. Regular exercise will also decrease blood sugar levels and improve glucose control. The most popular medication used for treatment is metformin, which works in various ways, including increasing the cells' sensitivity to insulin. In tablet form, it is a good candidate for medical storage.

Type 1 diabetes is more problematic, as many with this medical problem have large swings in their blood glucose levels. Regular monitoring of these levels and appropriate treatment with the right amount of insulin is necessary to remain healthy.

There are two common diabetic emergencies. These are related either to very low or very high glucose levels. If a diabetic, especially type 1, fails to eat regularly or takes too much insulin, they may develop hypoglycemia (low blood sugar). Hypoglycemia can occur very rapidly. Common symptoms are sweating, loss of coordination, confusion, and loss of consciousness.

In this case, a drink containing sugar will rapidly resolve the condition. Never give liquids to someone who is unconscious, however; the fluids could go down the respiratory passages, and suffocation could occur. If the patient is not mentally alert, place some sugar granules under his or her tongue. This will absorb rapidly without causing the tendency to choke.

On the other hand, very high glucose levels lead to diabetic ketoacidosis. This occurs as a result of missed insulin doses, chronically underdosed insulin, or both. Patients with this condition have a characteristic "fruity" odor to their breath. In addition to the usual symptoms, patients will experience nausea, vomiting, and abdominal pain. This is a major emergency that could lead to coma and even death. Small amounts of clear liquids are acceptable to give to someone with this condition, but without insulin and IV therapy, the prognosis is grave.

Insulin, like most liquid medications, will lose potency relatively soon after its expiration date. Because of the complexity of the manufacturing process, it is unlikely to be available in a collapse situation. What, then, can be done to maximize glucose control?

The goal should be to prevent complications, such as ketoacidosis. Diabetics will be unlikely to have perfect control off-grid, but it may be possible to keep their sugars below emergency levels. A period of less-than-optimal control may be survivable and might give some time for things to restabilize.

One therapeutic option is to stockpile the highest dose of metformin (oral diabetes medicine) in the hope that it may have some benefit in the insulin-deprived. Unfortunately, it will not make the pancreas produce insulin. A recent study suggests that metformin may be used along with insulin. In some diabetics, the addition of this drug resulted in lower amounts of insulin required for control. More study is warranted.

Another option is to regulate diet severely and subsist on a diet almost entirely comprised of protein and fats. The key is to restrict caloric intake significantly. This will be harmful in the long run, but frequent, small, high-protein meals may give the type 1 patient some time in a survival setting.

Type 2 diabetics (especially obese ones) may actually improve from the increased physical exertion and dietary restrictions that will be part and parcel of a long-term survival situation. An emphasis on limiting food intake to frequent small meals will be helpful here.

HIGH BLOOD PRESSURE

One of the most common chronic medical conditions is high blood pressure (hypertension). "Blood pressure" is the measure of the blood flow pushing against the walls of the arteries in your body. If this pressure is elevated over time, it can cause long-term damage. Many millions of adults in the United States have this condition, which is often asymptomatic (not noticeable). Because of this, it has been referred to as a "silent killer." Blood pressure tends to rise with increasing age and weight.

The medic should have, as part of his equipment, a stethoscope for listening and a sphygmomanometer (blood pressure cuff) to monitor blood pressure.

Blood pressure tends to vary at different times of the day and under different circumstances. Document at least three elevated pressures in a row before making the diagnosis. Readings above 160/100 are associated with higher frequency of complications. Persistent hypertension can lead to stroke, heart attack, heart failure, and chronic kidney failure. Commonly seen symptoms may include the following:

- ☤ Headaches
- ☤ Blurred vision
- ☤ Nausea and vomiting

Sometimes elevated pressures can damage a blood vessel in the brain. Strokes (cerebrovascular accidents, or CVAs) are bleeding episodes or clots in the brain that can occur as a high-pressure event and cause paralysis. The blood supply is interrupted, causing oxygen deficit in brain tissue.

A stroke is usually heralded by a sudden severe headache. Whatever functions are associated with the part of the brain affected will be lost or impaired. This might include the inability to speak, blindness, or loss of normal comprehension. Symptoms such as paralysis or weakness usually occur on only one side.

Although it may not be difficult to diagnose a major CVA in an austere setting, few options will exist for treating it. Blood thinners might help a stroke caused by a blockage due to a clot but worsen a stroke caused by a bleeding vessel. It could be difficult to tell which is which without advanced testing.

Keep the CVA victims on bed rest; sometimes, they may recover partial function after a period of time. If they do, most improvement will happen in the first few days.

Pregnancy-induced hypertension (re-eclampsia) is a serious condition that occurs late in a pregnancy. It may lead to seizures ("eclampsia") and blood clotting abnormalities. The first step to controlling elevated blood pressures is to return to a normal weight for your height and age. Most people who are overweight find that their blood pressure decreases (often back to normal) when they lose weight through dietary changes and exercise.

Dietary restriction of sodium is paramount in importance when it comes to decreasing pressures. Sodium is in just about everything you eat, so stop adding salt to food. Alcohol, nicotine, and perhaps, caffeine are also known to raise blood pressures, so avoiding these substances is an additional strategy. In a long-term survival situation, forced abstention may actually have a beneficial effect on overweight patients with hypertension.

The US National Institutes of Health (NIH) recommends the DASH (Dietary Approaches to Stop Hypertension) diet. A major feature of the plan is limiting intake of sodium and encouraging the consumption of nuts, whole grains, fish, poultry, fruits and vegetables while decreasing red meats, sweets, and sugar.

A number of medications with impressive names are available for the control of high blood pressure. Those with hypertension should be placed on one or more of these medications until their readings are back to normal. All of these commercially prepared products will be scarce in times of trouble.

Natural supplements have been used to help lower blood pressure, too. Any herb that has a sedative effect may also lower pressures. Valerian, passionflower, and lemon balm are some examples. Coenzyme Q10 has shown some promise in this field. Antioxidants, such as vitamin C and fish oil, may prevent free radicals from damaging artery walls.

Don't forget natural relaxation techniques. Meditation, yoga, and mild massage therapy should relax your patient and have a beneficial effect on their blood pressure.

Taking Blood Pressure

To use a sphygmomanometer, place the cuff around the upper arm and fill it up with air, using the attached bulb. Place your stethoscope over an area with a pulse (usually the crook of the arm) and listen while looking at the gauge on the cuff. Some new compact blood pressure units are meant to use on the wrist. With these, it is important to keep your wrist at the level of your heart when taking a reading.

When you take blood pressure, you are listening for the pulse to register on your stethoscope. Blood pressure is measured as systolic (blood pressure when the heart beats) and diastolic (blood pressure when the heart is at rest). Therefore, blood pressure is written down as systolic over diastolic; for example: (systolic pressure) 120 over 80 (diastolic pressure), written as 120/80.

Wherever the gauge is when you first hear the pulse is the systolic pressure. As the air deflates from the sphygmomanometer, the pulse will fade away. The point at which it first appears to fade is the diastolic pressure. You should be concerned with numbers that are above 140/90 in the supine or sitting position.

HEART DISEASE AND CHEST PAIN

Unlike in most medical books, we will not be spending a great deal of time discussing coronary artery disease, even though it is one of the leading causes of death in today's society. Why? Because of the loss of all the advances that have been made to deal with coronary disease, it would be difficult in a survival setting to do very much about heart attacks. We will have to accept that some folks with heart problems will do better than others.

Heart attacks (myocardial infarctions) involve the blockage of an artery that gives oxygen to a part of the heart muscle. That portion of the heart subsequently dies, either killing the patient or leaving them so incapacitated as to be unable to function. This decrease in function is most likely permanent. Men are most likely to have coronary artery disease, as female hormones seem to protect women, at least before menopause.

CPR may have limited value off-grid because of the lack of necessary advanced follow-up care that would be available. Despite this hard reality, it is still compulsory for any effective medic and how to perform it as described later in this book. Suspect a heart event if your patient experiences the following:

- A "crushing" sensation in the chest area
- Pain down the left arm
- Pain in the jaw area
- Weakness
- Fatigue
- Sweating
- Pale coloring

The main approach is to immediately give your patient a chewable adult aspirin (325 mg). This will act as a blood thinner, aiding in preventing further damage to the coronary artery and preserving oxygen flow. Aspirin can work within 15 minutes to prevent the formation of blood clots in people with known coronary artery disease or angina (cardiac-related chest pain).

A natural substance (capsaicin) found in cayenne pepper (at least 90,000 Scoville heat units, a measurement of perceived heat from spices) may also be helpful during a myocardial infarction. Give the conscious patient a glass of warm water mixed with 1 teaspoon of cayenne pepper. An alternative is to give two full droppers of cayenne pepper tincture or extract underneath the patient's tongue. Studies at the University of Cincinnati show an 85 percent decrease in cardiac cell death when cayenne pepper is given.

A person suffering a heart attack will feel most comfortable at a 45-degree angle, rather than lying flat. Complete rest will cause the least oxygen demand on the damaged heart. Loosen constrictive clothing, as tight clothes make a cardiac patient feel anxious and causes their damaged heart to beat faster, leading to more strain.

Aspirin, in small doses, is also reasonable as a preventative strategy. One baby aspirin (81 mg) daily is thought to help prevent the deposition of plaque inside the blood vessels. You might consider having all of your adults forty and over on this treatment.

Those in your group with coronary artery issues should stockpile whatever medications they take to deal with their symptoms. Angina can be treated with nitroglycerine tablets. Placed under the tongue, they will give rapid relief in most cases.

There are various other causes of chest pain. Injury to muscles and joints in the torso may mimic cardiac pain. This type of pain gets worse with movement of the affected area, and can be elicited by pressing on that area. Rest patients with angina and give them ibuprofen or acetaminophen for pain.

Chest pain is also seen in some patients with anxiety issues. This is usually accompanied by tremors, a rapid heart rate, and hyperventilation. Sedative herbs, such as valerian root, passion flower, and chamomile, may be helpful in this situation, as are some prescription medications, such as diazepam (Valium).

Acid reflux may also cause pain (usually burning in nature) in the chest area. This type of pain is usually improved with antacids in tablet form, such as calcium carbonate (Tums, Rolaids™, etc.) or liquid versions with magnesium hydroxide or aluminum hydroxide (Maalox, Mylanta™). Relaxation techniques, such as massage in a sitting position, may also help.

Ulcer and Acid Reflux Disease

Chronic stress, as will be seen in a survival setting, can manifest itself in both emotional and physical ways. One of the physical effects is increased stomach acid levels.

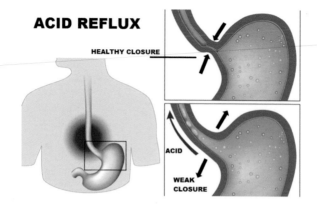

Excessive acid can cause an inflammation of the esophagus (the tube that goes from the throat to the stomach), the stomach itself, and the next part of the bowel (duodenum). The irritated lining weakens and forms an erosion (ulcer) and can cause bleeding or even perforate the entire thickness of the lining.

The major symptom of an ulcer is a burning or gnawing discomfort in the stomach area. This pain is often described as "heartburn." It usually occurs in the left or mid-upper abdomen or may travel up to the breastbone. Sometimes it is described as hunger pangs or indigestion.

To make the diagnosis of ulcer or acid reflux disease, the timing of the discomfort is important. Ulcer and acid reflux discomfort occurs soon after eating but is sometimes seen several hours after a meal. It can be differentiated from other causes of chest pain in another way: it gets better by drinking milk or taking antacids. As you can imagine, this wouldn't do much for angina.

Many ulcers and inflammation are caused by a bacterium, *Helicobacter pylori*. Antibiotics, such as amoxicillin and metronidazole, in combination are the most effective treatment for these ulcers.

Other causes include the overuse of ibuprofen or aspirin, which can be an irritant to the stomach in some people. Avoidance of these drugs can prevent these ulcers and inflammatory pain.

Acid reflux disease is caused by acid traveling up the esophagus. This is sometimes caused by an out-pouching at its base (hiatal hernia). The primary symptom is heartburn. It is usually relieved by antacids or by sleeping with the upper body raised.

Your patient may benefit from avoiding certain foods, including the following:

- Acidic fruit (for example, oranges)
- Fatty foods
- Coffee
- Certain teas
- Onions
- Peppermint
- Chocolate

Eating smaller meals and avoiding acidic foods before bedtime is a good strategy to prevent reflux. Chewing sugarless gum may also work. Obese individuals seem to suffer more from this problem, so weight loss might be helpful.

Medications that temporarily relieve acid reflux include calcium, magnesium, aluminum, and bismuth antacids, such as Tums, Maalox, Mylanta or Pepto-Bismol, as well as other medications, including ranitidine (Zantac™), cimetidine (Tagamet™), and omeprazole (Prilosec™). These medications are available in nonprescription strength and are easy to accumulate in quantity.

Home remedies abound for acid reflux, including the following:

Organic apple cider vinegar
Mix 1 tablespoon in 4 ounces of water and drink before each meal.

Aloe vera juice
Mix 1 ounce in 2 ounces of water and drink before a meal.

Baking soda
Mix 1 tablespoon in a glass of water and drink right away when you begin to feel heartburn.

Glutamine
An amino acid that has an anti-inflammatory effect and reduces acid reflux. It can be found in milk and eggs.

SEIZURE DISORDERS

Seizures occur when the brain's electrical system misfires. Instead of sending out signals in a controlled manner, a surge of haphazard energy goes through the brain. These abnormal signals can cause involuntary muscle contractions, poor control of certain organs, and loss of consciousness. A person with chronic convulsions is sometimes said to have "epilepsy."

Seizures may involve the entire brain or just one area. There are several types that have been identified, but we will concentrate on the most severe, a "grand mal" seizure. In grand mal seizures, you'll see violent shaking and jerking with loss of consciousness and bladder control. Strange sensations, known as "auras" (smells, colors, etc.), may herald an imminent convulsion.

There are various causes of convulsive disorders, such as the following:

- High fever (in children, mostly)
- Head injury
- Meningitis (infection of the central nervous system)
- Stroke
- Brain tumors
- Genetic predisposition
- Idiopathic (unknown—about 50 percent of cases)

Without modern medicine, we will have to watch for physical signs and symptoms to identify the problem. It is important to know that one seizure does not make someone an epileptic. In some cases (especially childhood seizures associated with fevers), a person might even outgrow the condition.

In addition to auras, there are triggers that sometimes cause a convulsion. A good example is a bright flashing light. Avoidance of these triggers will decrease the number of episodes.

The most important aspect of treatment when intravenous medication is no longer available will be to prevent the patient from injuring themselves during an attack. A tongue depressor with gauze taped around it and placed in the mouth was once a standard recommendation, but it was found to cause injuries to both the patient and the rescuer. Keep everything away from the patient's mouth, especially your fingers.

You shouldn't restrain the person physically, but remove nearby objects that could cause injury. An exception is if the patient is standing when the seizure starts. In this case, grab the patient and gently lower them to the floor. Placing them in the CPR "recovery" position (discussed in the CPR section of this book) will help keep their airway open.

Do not give oral fluids or medications to an epileptic after a seizure until they are fully awake and alert. A person who has had a seizure will tend to be difficult to rouse for a period of time. This "post-ictal" state will resolve on its own over time.

If the convulsion is caused by a fever, as in children, cool the patient down with wet compresses. Anyone in your survival group with a convulsive disorder should work towards stockpiling their medicine. Popular drugs are Dilantin, Tegretol™, valproic acid, and diazepam (Valium). Emphasize the importance of extra medications in cases of natural disaster or other emergencies.

Natural alternatives have long been espoused to decrease the frequency and severity of convulsions. Many vitamins and herbal supplements have a sedative effect, which calms the brain's electrical energy. They may be taken as a tea (1 teaspoon of the herb in 1 cup of water) or as a tincture (an extract with grain alcohol). The following are among those that have been reported as beneficial for prevention:

- Bacopa (*Bacopa monnieri*)
- Chamomile (*Matricaria recutita*)
- Kava (*Piper methysticum*—too much may damage the liver)
- Valerian (*Valeriana officinalis*)
- Lemon balm (*Melissa officinalis*)
- Passionflower (*Passiflora incarnata*)
- Vitamin B12 supplements
- Vitamin E supplements

When a Person Collapses

Sometimes, a patient may collapse, not from a convulsion but from simple fainting or head trauma. This person

- Will not have jerky spasms.
- Will usually regain alertness quickly.
- Will not lose control of their bladder.

Dehydration, overheating, low blood sugar and various other medical conditions can cause fainting. If someone feels as if they are about to collapse, they should sit down and put their head down between their knees to increase blood flow to the brain. If you see someone who is fainting from a standing position, grab them and gently lower them to the ground (in this case, on their back).

Evaluate the victim quickly. If someone has only fainted, they will be breathing and have a pulse. If this is the case, raise their legs about 12 inches off the ground and above the level of their heart and head. This will increase blood flow to the brain. Assess the patient for evidence of trauma, bleeding, or seizures. If so, treat as previously discussed in this book. If no pulse or breathing, begin CPR as discussed later.

Once a person who has fainted has been determined to be breathing, have a pulse, and have no bleeding injuries, tap on their shoulder and ask in a clear voice "Can you hear me?" or "Are you OK?" Loosen any obviously constricting clothing and make sure that they are getting lots of fresh air by keeping the area around them clear of crowds. If you are in an area that is hot, fan the patient or carefully carry them to a cooler area.

If you are successful in arousing the patient, ask them if they have any preexisting medical conditions, such as diabetes, heart disease, or epilepsy. Stay calm and speak in a reassuring manner. Don't let them get up for a period of time, even if they say that they are fine. People oftentimes are embarrassed and want to brush off the incident, but they are still at risk for another fall.

Once the victim is awake and alert (Do they know their name? Do they know where they are? What year it is?), you may slowly have the patient sit up if they are not otherwise injured. In normal times, call emergency medical personnel and wait until they arrive before having the patient stand up. If these aren't available, observe closely the rest of the day.

Common causes of fainting include dehydration and low blood sugar, so some oral intake may be helpful. Do this only if it is clear that they are completely conscious, alert, and able to function. Test their strength by having them raise their knees against the pressure of your hands. If they are weak, they should continue to rest. Close monitoring of the patient will be very important, as some internal injuries may not manifest for hours.

KIDNEY STONES AND GALL BLADDER DISEASE

The kidney and gall bladder are two organs that have the propensity in some people to develop an accumulation of crystals. These crystals form masses known as "stones." Some are large and some are as small as grains of sand, but any size can cause pain (sometimes excruciating). These issues can put group members out of commission at a time when they are most needed.

Kidney Stones

Kidney stones are most commonly seen in people who fail to keep themselves well hydrated. Even small stones can lead to significant pain (renal colic), and the larger ones can cause blockages that can disrupt the function of the organ. Once you have had a kidney stone, it is likely you will get them again at one point or another. Kidney stones are usually not associated with infections.

Once formed in the kidney, stones usually do not cause symptoms until they begin to move down the tubes

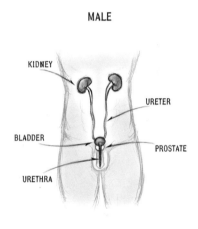

MALE

KIDNEY

URETER

BLADDER

PROSTATE

URETHRA

URINARY SYSTEM

that connect the kidneys to the bladder (the ureters). When this happens, the stones can block the flow of urine. This causes swelling of the kidney affected as well as significant pain. Kidney stones as small as grains of sand may reach the bladder without incident and then cause pain as they attempt to pass through the tube that goes from the bladder to the outside (the urethra).

There are several different types of kidney stones:

- **Calcium stones.** The most common, they occur more often in men than in women, usually in those 20–40 years old. Calcium can combine with other substances, such as oxalate, phosphate, or carbonate, to form a stone.

- **Cysteine stones.** These form in people who have cysteinuria, a condition that tends to run in families.
- **Struvite stones.** This variety is mostly found in women and can grow quite large. They can cause blockages at any point in the urinary tract. Frequent and chronic infections are a risk factor.
- **Uric acid stones.** More common in men than in women, these stones are associated with conditions such as gout.

To diagnose a kidney stone, look for pain that starts suddenly and comes and goes. Pain is commonly felt on the side of the back (the flank). Lightly pounding on the right and left flank at the level of the lowest rib will cause significant pain in patients with kidney stones or kidney infections. As the stone moves, so will the pain; it will travel down the abdomen and could settle in the groin or even the urethral area.

Other symptoms of renal stones can include the following:

- Bloody urine
- Fever and chills
- Nausea and vomiting

Some dietary changes may prevent the formation of kidney stones, especially if they are made of calcium. Avoid foods such as the following:

- Spinach
- Rhubarb
- Beets
- Parsley
- Sorrel
- Chocolate

Decreasing dairy intake is another step to take, as this will restrict the amount of calcium available for stone formation, keeping them as small as possible and, therefore, easier to pass.

Your treatment goal as medical provider is to assist the stone to pass through the system quickly. Have your patient drink at least 8 glasses of water per day to produce a large amount of urine. The flow will help move the stone along. Cranberry juice is very helpful, as well; one advantage is that it does not deplete the body of potassium, while diuretics such as furosemide (Lasix™) and hydrochlorothiazide (HCTZ) often do.

Pain relievers can help control the pain of passing the stones (renal colic). For most pain, ibuprofen will be the available treatment of choice. Stronger pain medications, if you can get them, may be necessary for severe cases.

Some of the larger stones will be chronic issues, as the technology and surgical options used to remove these will not be available in a collapse scenario. Medications specific to the type of stone may be helpful. The following decrease the likelihood of formation of uric acid stones:

- Allopurinol (prescription medicine for uric acid stones and gout)
- Antibiotics (for struvite stones)
- Sodium bicarbonate or sodium citrate (which increases the alkalinity of the urine)

A good home remedy to relieve discomfort and aid passage of the stone is lemon juice, olive oil, and apple cider vinegar. With the first twinge of pain, drink a mixture of 2 ounces of lemon juice and 2 ounces of olive oil. Then, drink a large glass of water. After 1 hour, drink a mixture of 1 tablespoon of raw apple cider vinegar with 2 ounces of lemon juice in a large glass of water. Repeat this process every 1–2 hours until improved.

Other natural substances that may help:

- Horsetail tea (a natural diuretic)
- Pomegranate juice
- Dandelion root tea
- Celery tea
- Basil tea

Gall Bladder Stones

The gall bladder is a sac-like organ that is attached to the liver; it stores the bile that the liver secretes. Gallstones are firm deposits that form inside the gallbladder and could block the passage of bile. This blockage can cause a great deal of pain and inflammation (cholecystitis).

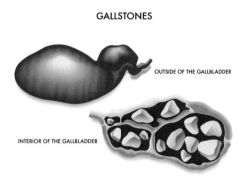

GALLSTONES

OUTSIDE OF THE GALLBLADDER

INTERIOR OF THE GALLBLADDER

There are two main types of gallstones:

Cholesterol stones—The grand majority, these are not related to the actual cholesterol levels in the bloodstream.

Bilirubin stones—These occur in those people who have illnesses that destroy their red blood cells. The byproducts of this destruction releases a substance (bilirubin) into the bile and forms a stone.

Risk factors for gallstones include obesity, female gender (especially if they have had children), and age over forty. Additional risk factors include diabetes, chronic liver disease, and low blood counts (anemia).

Luckily, most people with gallstones don't have any symptoms. If a large stone causes a blockage, however, they may experience biliary colic. Symptoms of biliary colic include the following:

- Cramping right upper abdomen pain (spreading to the back)
- Fever
- Jaundice (yellowing of the skin and whites of the eyes)
- Discolored bowel movements (gray or grayish-white)
- Nausea and vomiting

The classical finding on physical examination is "Murphy's sign." Press with one hand just below the midline of the lowest rib on the front right. Then, ask your patient to breathe deeply. If the gallbladder is tender, the patient should complain of significant pain at the site.

Unfortunately, the main treatment for gallstones is to surgically remove the gallbladder (which you can live without and stay healthy). As surgical suites are unlikely to be available in a collapse situation, you might consider some alternative remedies. The following are mostly preventative measures:

- Apple cider vinegar (mixed with apple juice)
- Chanca piedra, a plant that is native to the Amazon; translated, the name means "break stones."
- Peppermint
- Turmeric
- Alfalfa

- Ginger root
- Dandelion root
- Artichoke leaves
- Beet, carrot, grape, lemon juices

Sadly, it is very difficult to eliminate most of the risk factors for gallbladder disease. If you're forty, female, and have children, there is not much you can do about it. Dietary changes to decrease intake of high-cholesterol foods may be helpful.

VIII.

✚ ✚ ✚

OTHER IMPORTANT MEDICAL ISSUES

CPR IN AUSTERE SETTINGS

Most medical books start off with a chapter on cardio-pulmonary resuscitation, so you might wonder why this subject has not been given coverage so far in this volume. The answer is based on hard realities that we must confront in a survival scenario.

Although CPR is an important skill that everyone should know, there are fewer situations in a collapse scenario where it will return a victim to normal function. There are only a small number of circumstances where a patient goes from being a patient in need of resuscitation to a person who is back to normal.

CPR is best used as a stabilization strategy. You want to get the heart pumping and breathing supported so that you can get your patient as quickly as possible to a facility where there are ventilators, defibrillators, and other high technology. But what about a situation where this technology is no longer available?

There won't be cardiac bypasses for your patient who has had a heart attack. There won't be surgical suites for your patient with a shotgun blast to the abdomen or chest. The sobering truth is that many of these injuries will be mortal wounds. This means that death is the inevitable end result, no matter what you try to do. The poor prognosis for these people in hard times is tragic; it makes you truly appreciate the benefits of modern medicine.

There are still instances, however, where CPR may actually restore a gravely ill person to normal function. Airway obstruction by a foreign object can be dealt with by using the Heimlich maneuver. Environmental conditions, such as hypothermia, heat stroke, or smoke inhalation, will often respond to resuscitative efforts with complete recovery. Severe anaphylactic reactions may require CPR until the patient responds to epinephrine (EpiPen) and resolves the attack. Rarer events, such as lightning strikes or drowning, may require resuscitation to revive the victim.

I chose not to put a large number of illustrations or an entire course on how to do CPR in this book. There is no substitution for learning it in person by taking a hands-on course, mandatory for anyone who expects to be a caregiver in a long-term survival scenario.

Airway Obstruction

One situation where you can save a life by knowing how to perform a simple maneuver is in the case of an airway obstruction. This most commonly occurs as a result of food lodging in the back of the throat and cutting off respiration.

If you see a conscious adult in sudden respiratory distress, ask quickly, "Are you choking on something?" If they can answer you, there is still air passing into their lungs. If it's a complete blockage, they will be unable to speak. They will probably be agitated and holding their throat, but they will hear you and (frantically) nod their head "yes." Quick action will be necessary.

Tell the victim that you're there to help them and immediately get into position for the Heimlich maneuver, otherwise known as an "abdominal thrust." Get behind the victim and make a fist with your right hand. Place your fist above the belly button; then, wrap your left arm around the patient and grasp the right fist. Make sure your arms are positioned just below the ribcage. With a forceful upward motion, press your fist abruptly into the abdomen. You might have to do this multiple times before you dislodge the foreign body.

If your patient loses consciousness and you are unable to dislodge the obstructive item, place the patient in a supine position and straddle them across the thighs or hips. Open their mouth and make sure that the object can't be removed manually. Give several upward abdominal thrusts with the heels of your palms above the belly button (one hand on top of the other). Check again; you might have partially dislodged the offending morsel of food.

In old movies, you might see someone slap the victim hard on the back; this is unlikely to dislodge a foreign object and will waste precious time. An exception to this is in an infant: Place the baby over your forearm (facing down) and apply several blows with the heel of your hand to the upper back.

An extreme method that can be used to open an airway is the tracheotomy. This procedure, also called a cricothyroidotomy, involves cutting an opening in the windpipe below the level of an obstruction. Tracheotomy should be performed only when an airway obstruction completely prevents the ability to breathe after multiple Heimlich maneuvers have been unsuccessful.

To perform a tracheotomy, you will need a sharp blade and some sort of tube, even a straw. Don't worry about antiseptics for now; you are performing this procedure because someone may die in the next few minutes.

The procedure goes as follows:

1. Start at the Adam's apple. Move about 1 inch down the neck until you feel a bulge. This is the cricoid cartilage.
2. Make a horizontal incision with a knife or a razor blade in the crease between the Adam's apple and the cricoid cartilage. This incision can be less than 1 inch long.
3. Incise downward ½-inch deep or so. There shouldn't be a lot of blood.
4. Below the incision, you'll see the greyish crico-thyroid membrane. Make an incision through it; this should enable passage of air into the lungs. Be careful not to cut too deeply.
5. Place something hollow in the opening 1 inch deep, to maintain a clear airway. A straw would do in a pinch. Try to get it a couple of inches down the windpipe; doing this makes it less likely to fall out.
6. If the patient fails to breathe on their own, you may need to perform CPR, including rescue breaths through the tube you inserted.

This obviously is a dangerous procedure. A lot can go wrong, but the patient is dying and it may be your last resort. Only consider it when help is *not* on the way, and you have tried every other option first.

CPR in the Unconscious Patient

If you come across someone who is apparently unconscious, be certain to first verify their mental status. Simply ask them loudly, "Are you OK?" No answer? Grasp the person's shoulders and move them gently while continuing to ask them questions. If they are still unresponsive, it's time to check their pulse and respiration. If they aren't breathing or no pulse is felt, it's time to start resuscitative efforts:

1. Place your patient in a position so that they are lying flat on their back.
2. Begin chest compressions by placing the heel of your hand in the middle of the chest palm down, over the lower half of the breastbone at the nipple level.

3. Place your other hand on top and interlace your fingers.
4. Position yourself directly above your hands (arms straight) and press downward in such a fashion that the breastbone (sternum) is compressed about 2 inches. You would want less pressure in a child.
5. Allow the chest to recoil completely. Perform 30 compressions at a rate of at least 100 per minute. Be certain to avoid the rib cage, as broken ribs are a common complication of the procedure.

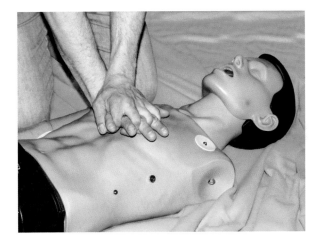

After 30 chest compressions, evaluate the victim for breathing and clear the airway. Look quickly inside the mouth for a foreign object. If there is none, place the patient's head in a position that will enable the clearest passage for air to enter the body. This is called the "chin lift." Tilt the head back (unless there is evidence of a neck injury); grasp the underside of the chin and lower jaw with one hand and lift. Using this method, the tongue and other throat structures are placed in a position that helps the patient take in oxygen. A useful medical device in this situation is an airway. There are both rigid oral and flexible nasal versions that help keep the patient's airway open.

If you aren't trained in CPR, just continue compressions. If you *do* know CPR, you may give 2 long breaths mouth-to-mouth (3–5 seconds between each one). These are called "rescue breaths." Pinch the nose closed to prevent the escape of air that needs to get into the lungs.

You can determine the effectiveness of your efforts by watching the patient's chest rise as you give the breaths. Continue giving 30 compressions, then 2 rescue breaths for 5 cycles or 2 minutes. Then, check your patient's status. Once you have started CPR, don't stop until the patient has responded or it is clear that they will not.

Many people are reluctant to perform rescue breaths because of concerns about contagious disease. If this is an issue, take a nitrile glove and cut the ends off the two middle fingers. Place over the victim's mouth (cut glove fingers down) as you breathe for them. This provides a barrier that still enables air flow. Commercially produced protective CPR masks are also available.

Another useful item for your medical supplies is a bag valve mask, otherwise known by the brand name Ambu™ bag. This can be placed on the patient's mouth to form a seal through which you can ventilate them by pressing on an air-filled "bag." This will force air into the respiratory passages.

After 30 minutes of CPR without result, the pupils of the patient's eyes will likely be dilated and not respond to light. At this point, your patient has expired and you can cease your efforts. Some may feel this is not long; in truth, however, just a few minutes without oxygen are enough to cause irreversible brain damage. In a grid-down situation, you will not be equipped to provide long-term chronic care to someone who no longer has brain activity.

There are units known as defibrillators available that, though quite expensive, may be useful in a cardiac arrest. These machines produce an electric shock to the heart and sometimes can restart a pulse that has stopped. If caused by a heart attack, a patient suffering a cardiac arrest without defibrillation will have a very low survival rate.

"Home" defibrillators can be found online and are surprisingly easy to use:

1. Turn the unit on and connect the electrodes per the instructions.
2. Place one electrode pad on the right chest above the nipple and below the collarbone.
3. Place the other on the left chest outside the nipple and several inches below the armpit. The unit will analyze the heart rate (or lack of one) and tell you whether a shock is necessary.
4. If a shock is indicated, clear everyone away from the patient and press the button to activate the electric shock.
5. Recheck vital signs and begin chest compressions as needed.

If you are successful in establishing a pulse and breathing in your unconscious patient and, for some reason, you must leave them, position them so that they will not vomit and possibly aspirate stomach acid into the lungs (see image below). This is known as the "recovery position."

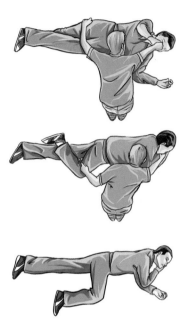

The recovery position

To achieve the recovery position, take the following steps:

1. Kneel on one side facing the patient.
2. Position the patient's arm (the one closest to you) perpendicular to the body.
3. Flex the elbow.
4. Position the other arm across the body.
5. Bend the leg that is farthest from you up; reach behind the knee and pull the thigh toward you.
6. Use your other arm to pull the shoulder farthest from you while rolling the body toward you.
7. Maintain the upper leg in a flexed position so that the body is stabilized.

As we stated above, although CPR will be of limited use when modern medical facilities are not available, it is still important to know. A survival medic should not only be skilled in performing CPR, but should also teach it to every group member.

HEADACHE

Headaches are one of the most common medical symptoms that you will see in your role as medic. Although there are almost more causes for headaches than you can reasonably write down, in a survival setting, it's good to know the common causes are:

- Hunger
- Dehydration
- Stress
- Infections
- Fevers
- Elevated blood pressure
- Caffeine or alcohol withdrawal
- Fumes

Headaches that occur suddenly may be related to infection, especially in the ears or sinuses, colds, or flus, but may also herald a life-threatening event, such as a stroke.

Headache Types

Tension headache

By far, the most frequently seen type of headache is the tension headache. This is caused by spasms of the muscles of the neck and head. Tension headache is usually seen bilaterally (on both sides) and in the back of the head, neck, or both. They may be related to stress, anxiety or depression, a head injury, or even just time spent with the head or neck in an abnormal position. A sensation of pressure or tightening is the most common symptom.

This type of headache may be improved by massaging the back of the neck and temples. Ibuprofen and acetaminophen are old standbys as treatment. Identifying the situation that triggers the headache may help avoid future episodes.

Sinus headache

Sinus headaches are often caused by infections. They are associated with constant pain in the front of the face. A sinus is an air-filled cavity in the bones of the skull. The forehead, cheeks, or the bridge of the nose are the areas affected most by sinus infections; they often may be one-sided, which will help you to make the diagnosis. Sudden head movement may intensify the pain.

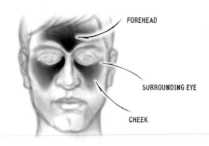

SINUS HEADACHE

To treat headaches caused by sinusitis, amoxicillin (veterinary equivalent: Fish Mox Forte), 500 mg – times a day for a week, is a reasonable first choice. If you are allergic to the penicillin family of drugs, consider sulfamethoxazole/trimethoprim (veterinary equivalent: Bird Sulfa), either 160 mg or 800 mg (as needed) twice daily. Nasal decongestants, such as pseudoephedrine (Sudafed), may give some relief; so may sterile saline nasal rinses.

Migraines

Migraine headaches are common. The exact cause of migraines is uncertain but may be related to spasms in the blood vessels. Women are more susceptible than men.

A specific pattern of symptoms is seen in this variety of headache:

- Pain behind the eye (usually one-sided)
- Sensitivity to light, noise or odors
- Nausea and vomiting (causing loss of appetite or stomach discomfort)
- Vision changes (blurring, light and color phenomena)

Bed rest in the dark will be helpful here, as well as ibuprofen or acetaminophen. Some migraine medications use caffeine, which can be effective. Teas and coffee might be alternatives in an austere setting. If you are a chronic migraine sufferer, ask your physician for sumatriptan (Imitrex™), a strong anti-migraine medication, to stockpile.

Less common causes of headache include a serious infection of the central nervous system (meningitis). Along with headaches, meningitis presents with a stiff neck, fever, and possibly a rash. This condition may be caused by bacteria, viruses, or even fungi. You could treat this condition with antibiotics and antivirals but expect variable results.

Uncontrolled high blood pressure or a burst blood vessel in the brain may cause a stroke. Besides the sudden onset of a severe headache, the patient may lose strength in the arm and leg on one side, have decreased motion on one side of the face, and absent or slurred speech.

Natural Headache Relief

If you would like a strategy to deal with a headache without drugs, try the following:

- Place an ice pack where the headache is.
- Have someone massage the back of your neck.
- Using two fingers, apply rotating pressure where the headache is.
- Lie down in a dark, quiet room. Get some sleep if at all possible. If your blood pressure is elevated, lay on your left side (pressure is usually lowest in this position).
- Track what you were doing or perhaps what you ate before the headache started; avoid that activity or food if possible.

A number of herbal remedies are available that might help headache. Feverfew is an herb that may decrease blood vessel constriction and is anti-inflammatory. This can be taken on a daily basis (1–2 leaves) for those with chronic problems. (*Warning: don't use feverfew during pregnancy or nursing.*) Gingko biloba has a similar action. For external use, consider lavender or rosemary oil. Massage each temple with 1–2 drops every few hours.

The pain of tension headaches can be relieved if you use herbs that have sedative and antispasmodic properties. Teas made from valerian, skullcap, lemon balm, and passionflower have both. Herbal muscle relaxants may also help; rosemary, chamomile, and mint teas are popular options.

EYE ISSUES

By picking up this book, you have demonstrated that you have excellent foresight. Unfortunately, that doesn't mean that you necessarily have excellent eyesight. Human beings aren't perfect, and one of our most common imperfections is that of being nearsighted (having myopia) or farsighted (having hyperopia).

Most of us correct our eye issues with eyeglasses or contact lenses. In a survival setting, these vision aids become more precious than gold, but most people haven't made provision for replacement pairs in their storage. I can't think of anything scarier than being on your own and not being able to see. Therefore, your medical supplies should have multiple pairs. You might even consider corrective eye surgery (laser-assisted in situ keratomileusis, or LASIK). It is highly successful and one of the safest surgical procedures in existence.

Eye-protection glasses are another required item. Many of us with perfect vision will be negligent about wearing eye protection when we chop wood or other chores likely to be part of off-grid living. Without eye protection, the risk of injury when performing some strenuous tasks will be much higher.

Most people don't consider sunglasses to be a medical supply item, but they are. Even if you are just taking a hike outdoors, sunglasses provide eye protection from ultraviolet light. UV light causes, over time, damage to the retinal cells, which can lead to a clouding over of your eye's lenses (cataracts). This condition can only be repaired by surgery that will not be available in a collapse. Protection from UV light helps prevent long-term damage.

Sunglasses may also prevent a type of vision loss known as "snow blindness" (photokeratitis), a burning of the cornea that comes from overexposure to UV light. This is painful and dangerous in the wilderness, but, luckily, will go away on its own if the affected eye is covered with a patch. Bottom line: Whenever you are outdoors, you should ask yourself why you *aren't* wearing eye protection.

Infections of the Eye

There are various eye conditions that will be more common in a grid-down situation. The most common will be conjunctivitis (pinkeye).

Conjunctivitis is an inflammation that causes the affected eye to become red and itchy, and many times will cause a milky discharge. It can be caused by chemical irritation, a foreign body, an allergy, or an infection.

Pinkeye is highly contagious among children because of their habit of rubbing their eyes and then touching other people or items. While children may do it more than adults, studies have shown that people of all ages commonly touch their faces and eyes with their (often dirty) hands throughout the day.

Irritated red eyes with tears may also be seen in allergic reactions, which can be treated with antihistamines orally or antihistamine eye drops. Eye allergies can be differentiated from eye infections in that eye allergies are less likely to have a milky discharge associated with them.

To avoid spreading the germs that can cause eye infections, do the following:

- Don't share eye drops with others.
- Don't touch the tip of a bottle of eye drops with your hands or your eyes, because that can contaminate it with germs. Keep the bottle 3 inches above your eye.
- Don't share eye makeup with others.
- Never put contact lenses in your mouth to wet them. Many bacteria and viruses—maybe even the virus that causes cold sores (herpes)—are present in your mouth and could easily spread to your eyes.
- Change your contacts often. The longer they stay in your eyes, the higher the chance is that your eye can get infected.
- Wash your hands regularly.

Antibiotics such as doxycycline, 100 mg twice a day for a week, will relieve infectious conjunctivitis. To treat pinkeye using natural products, pick one or more of the following methods:

- Apply a wet chamomile or goldenseal tea bag to the closed, affected eye for 10 minutes every 2 hours.
- Make a strong chamomile (*Euphrasia officinalis*; also known as eyebright) tea. Let it cool and use the liquid as an eyewash (using an eyecup) 3–4 times daily.
- Use 1 teaspoon of baking soda in 2 cups of cool water as an eyewash solution.

- Dissolve 1 tablespoon of honey in 1 cup hot water; let cool and use as eyewash.
- Use any of the solutions described above on gauze or cloth, and then apply a compress to the affected eye for 10 minutes every 2 hours. Placing a slice of cucumber over the eyes can cool them, providing relief.

Another common eye issue is a sty, essentially a pimple which has formed on the eyelid. It causes redness and some swelling and is generally uncomfortable. Warm, moist compresses are helpful in enabling the sty to drain. Any of the previously mentioned antibiotic or natural treatments for conjunctivitis can also be used.

Eye Trauma

The great majority of eye injuries are avoidable with a little planning. Despite this, it is likely you will come upon an eye injury at one point or another. Here are just a few of the ways eye injuries occur:

- Accidents while using tools
- Spatter from bleach or other household chemicals
- Hedge clippers or lawn mowers
- Grease splatter from cooking
- Chopping wood

Whenever anyone presents to you with eye pain, do a careful examination. A foreign object is the most likely cause of the problem. Use a moist cotton swab (Q-tip) to lift and evert the eyelid. This will enable you to effectively examine the area. An amount of clean water can be used as irrigation to flush out the foreign object. Alternatively, touch the object lightly with the Q-tip to dislodge it.

After ensuring that there is no foreign object still present, look at the cornea, the clear layer of tissue over the iris (the colored part of the eye). The cornea protects the eye and helps with focusing. Damage to this layer of tissue, called a "corneal abrasion," may be caused by any of the things listed earlier; people who wear contact lenses are especially at risk. The patient will probably relate to you that they feel as if there's a grain of sand in their eye.

After cleaning the eye out with water and using antibiotic eye drops (if available), cover the closed eye with an eye pad and tape. Ibuprofen is useful for pain relief. Over the next few days, the eye should heal.

Occasionally, blunt trauma to the eye or even simple actions such as coughing or sneezing may cause a patch of blood to appear in the white of the eye. This is a subconjunctival hemorrhage (or hyphema) and certainly can be alarming to the patient. Luckily, this type of hemorrhage is not dangerous, and will go away on its own without any treatment. If there is a loss of vision associated with the hyphema, however, there *is* cause for concern. Evaluate this injury as described for abrasions. Keeping the patient's head elevated will enable any blood to drain to the lower part of the eye chamber. This strategy may help preserve vision.

NOSEBLEEDS

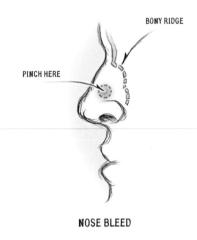

BONY RIDGE

PINCH HERE

NOSE BLEED

It's a rare individual who has never had a nosebleed. The nose has many tiny blood vessels and is situated in a vulnerable position because it protrudes from the face.

Nosebleeds can occur from outside causes, such as trauma to the face, or by factors that affect the inside of the nose, such as excessive "picking" or irritation from upper respiratory infections. Environmental factors, such as cold or dry climates, may also play a role. In rare cases, underlying illness, such as faulty blood clotting, may be implicated.

Do the following to effectively stop a nosebleed in a patient:

1. Have the patient sit upright with their head tipped slightly forward. Although you may have been taught to tilt your patient's head backward, this may just cause blood to run down the back of the throat.
2. Have the patient breathe through their mouth.
3. Using your thumb and index finger, firmly pinch the soft part of the nose just below the bone. Push towards the face. Spray the nose with a medicated nasal spray, such as oxymetazoline hydrochloride, 0.05 percent (Afrin), before applying pressure.
4. Apply an ice pack to the side that is bleeding. Cold constricts the blood vessels and may help stop the bleeding.
5. Apply pressure for 5–10 minutes. Be patient.
6. Check to see if your patient's nose is still bleeding after 10 minutes. If still bleeding, hold it for 10 more minutes.
7. Place a little petroleum jelly inside the nose.

In prolonged cases, a strip cut from gauze impregnated with Celox or QuikClot may be placed delicately in the nose with blunt tweezers or a Kelly clamp. Alternatively, the bleeding nostril can be flushed with sterile saline; then, gently introduce a thin strip of cloth drenched in epinephrine (from an EpiPen or other anaphylactic shock kit) gently into the nostril. Do not remove the packing for several hours. Other commercial products, such as NasalCEASE™ or WoundSeal, are available and are thought to be effective; you should consider them as medical storage items.

Whether the bleeding is due to trauma or not, blowing the nose to eject blood and clots should be avoided, as it may restart the bleeding.

The "Broken" Nose

What is usually referred to as a "broken" nose consists of either an actual fracture of the delicate bones that connect the nose to the rest of the skull, or just damage to the cartilage in the nose. If the nose bones are fractured, the patient will find that any pressure on the nose is very painful. Although it may be painful, an obvious deformity of the nose due to trauma can possibly be adjusted back into place.

Damage to the cartilage may also cause deformity and difficult breathing due to swelling. You may choose to reduce the deformity by using both hands to straighten the cartilage. This may be appropriate as the injured nose, if deformed, will not straighten out by itself. Be aware that this may cause further damage.

You might then consider taping the nose in its normal position. Place some ice wrapped in a cloth over the nose for periods of 20 minutes, taking breaks in between to avoid damage from the cold, throughout the next 48 hours to reduce swelling and discomfort. Acetaminophen and ibuprofen will also be helpful in this circumstance. Swelling in nasal passages may be improved with a nasal decongestant.

EARACHE

It's a rare parent who hasn't had to deal with this problem in their child at one point or another. In some cases, it's a chronic problem that affects the quality of life of an otherwise healthy child. The most common symptom relating to the ear is pain, usually due to an infection.

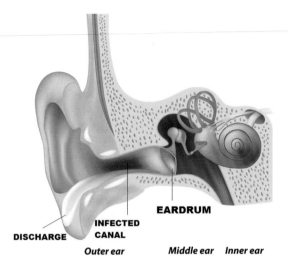

EARDRUM

INFECTED CANAL

DISCHARGE

Outer ear   *Middle ear*   *Inner ear*

The ear is divided into three chambers: the outer ear, middle ear, and inner ear. The most common ear infections will be in the external and middle ear chambers.

The easiest way to prevent ear infections is to carefully use cotton swabs moistened with rubbing alcohol to dry the ear canal after swimming or excessive sweating. Forceful use of a cotton swab, however, is to be avoided; normally, you shouldn't place anything in the ear canal smaller than your elbow.

Ear Infections

Otitis Externa

Inflammation of the ear is called "otitis." Otitis externa, also known as "swimmer's ear," is an infection of the outer ear canal, and most commonly affects children aged 4–14 years old. Cases peak during summer months, when most people go swimming. Bacteria will accumulate and multiply in water or sweat. Once caught in the ear canal, inflammation and discomfort ensue.

Symptoms of otitis externa include the following:

- ☙ Gradual development of an earache or, possibly, itching
- ☙ Pain worsened by pulling on the ear
- ☙ Ringing in the ears (tinnitus) or decreased hearing
- ☙ A "full" sensation in the ear canal, with swelling and redness
- ☙ Thick drainage from the ear canal

Standard treatment may include a warm compress to the ear to help with pain control. An antibiotic or steroidal ear drop will be useful, and should be applied for 7 days. To get the most effect from the medicine, place the drops in the ear with the patient lying on their side (the opposite one from the affected ear). They should stay in that position for 5 minutes to completely coat the ear canal. Severe cases may be treated with oral antibiotics (such as amoxicillin) and ibuprofen.

Otitis Media

The most common cause of earache is an infection of the middle ear, otitis media. When visualized with an otoscope (a scope for examining the ear canal), the eardrum is normally shiny and grayish. When there is an infection in the middle ear canal, the eardrum will appear dull. This is because there is pus or inflammatory fluid behind it. Standard treatment often includes oral antibiotics and ibuprofen, especially in adults with the infection.

Otitis media is most common, however, in infants and toddlers. This is why mothers are always cautioned against bottle or breast-feeding with their baby lying flat. You can expect one or more of the following with otitis media:

- ☙ Pain, more so when lying down
- ☙ Difficulty sleeping, and irritability
- ☙ Fever
- ☙ Loss of appetite
- ☙ Loss of balance
- ☙ Holding or pulling the affected ear
- ☙ Drainage of fluid from the affected ear
- ☙ Difficulty hearing from the affected ear

A number of natural remedies are available for earache. Try the following procedure:

1. Mix rubbing alcohol and vinegar in equal quantities, or alternatively, hydrogen peroxide.
2. Place 3–4 drops into affected ear.
3. Wait 5 minutes; then, tilt head to drain out the mixture.
4. Use plain warm olive oil and place 2–3 drops into the ear canal. A cotton ball with 2 drops of eucalyptus oil may be secured to the ear opening during sleep.

Other Ear Problems

Inner-ear canal issues, including inflammation (otitis interna), often cause dizziness (vertigo). These patients commonly feel nauseous as well as dizzy. Treatment with dimenhydrinate (Dramamine™) can help with symptoms. Amoxicillin (veterinary equivalent: Fish Mox Forte), 500 mg 3 times a day for 7 days, is an appropriate antibiotic therapy if the otitis was caused by an infection.

Ear wax (cerumen) is a chronic problem for certain people. Cerumen is normal and protective in healthy ears. It traps dust particles before they can reach the ear drum.

Normally, people use cotton swabs to remove ear wax, but this method often pushes ear wax farther in. Cleaning the opening of the ear canal with a twisted, moist washcloth is safer.

When, for whatever reason, cerumen is lodged against the eardrum, it can affect hearing. Other symptoms include the following:

- Earache
- Hearing loss
- Itching
- Odor or discharge
- Ringing in the ear (tinnitus)

Commercial ear rinses with special syringes are available for treatment. Standard home remedies involve a few drops of mineral or baby oil in the ear. This softens the wax, which can then be flushed out with 3 percent hydrogen peroxide. Some people just use the hydrogen peroxide by itself.

HEMORRHOIDS

Hemorrhoids are painful, swollen veins in the lower portion of the rectum that often protrude from the anus. A likely cause is low dietary fiber, which leads to hard stools. This causes straining during bowel movements. Hemorrhoids are extremely common during pregnancy.

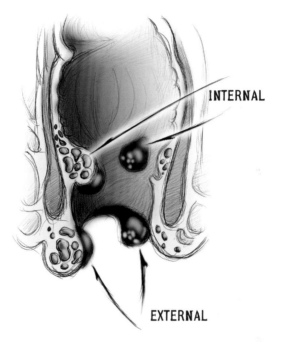

INTERNAL

EXTERNAL

HEMORRHOIDS

Hemorrhoids are asymptomatic unless they develop a clot and become inflamed (thrombosis), which will cause constant pain and may even make it difficult to sit down.

Hemorrhoids may be internal or external. Symptoms include the following:

- ⚕ Anal itching
- ⚕ Bleeding, usually seen on toilet tissue
- ⚕ Pain, which is worse in the sitting position
- ⚕ Pain during bowel movements
- ⚕ Painful bumps near the anus

Diagnosis is made simply by looking at the area. Hemorrhoids will appear as bluish lumps at the edge of the anal opening. If the hemorrhoid is internal, the diagnosis is made through a rectal exam with a gloved finger.

Hemorrhoids only require treatment when symptomatic. Treatments for hemorrhoids include the following:

- Mild corticosteroid creams, such as Anusol HC™, or wipes, such as Tucks™ pads, to help reduce pain and swelling.
- Stool softeners to decrease further trauma to the inflamed tissue.
- Witch hazel compresses to reduce itching.
- Warm water baths (sitz baths) to reduce general discomfort.

Even painful hemorrhoids will usually go away by themselves over a few weeks, but sometimes the discomfort is so severe that you may be required to remove the clot from the swollen vein. This is performed by incising the skin over the hemorrhoid and draining the clotted blood.

A scalpel may be used (preferably under local anesthesia) to incise the hemorrhoid after cleaning the area thoroughly with Betadine. Cut just deep enough to evacuate the clot. The patient should experience quick relief as a result. Gauze pads should be placed at the site to absorb any bleeding. In rare cases, a suture may be needed.

It should be noted that this procedure is not the best way to remove a hemorrhoid, as simple incision does not remove it in its entirety. It may come back at a later time. Modern procedures, such as placing bands around the hemorrhoid, are less traumatic and more permanent in their results.

BIRTH CONTROL, PREGNANCY, AND DELIVERY

It's a rare individual who doesn't have a wife, girlfriend, mother, daughter or granddaughter that isn't of childbearing age (13–50 years old). In a long-term disaster, society will be unstable and organized medical care will be spotty at best, nonexistent at worst. One of the least welcome events might be one that, for many families, is ordinarily considered a blessing: a pregnancy.

A pregnancy and the possible complications that accompany it will be a burden in a disaster. A pregnant woman will be at less than 100 percent efficiency at the exact wrong time, and complications could occur.

The death rate among pregnant women (also known as the maternal mortality rate) at the time of the American Revolution was about 2–4 percent *per pregnancy*. Given that the average woman in the year 1800 could expect 6–10 pregnancies over the course of her reproductive life, the cumulative maternal mortality rate easily approached 25 percent. That means that one out of four women died from complications of being pregnant, either early, during the childbirth, or even soon after a successful delivery.

If a major disaster occurs, women might face unacceptable levels of risk. There won't be either medicine or medical supplies in which to treat pregnancy and childbirth complications. Deaths may happen simply because there are no IV fluids or medications to stop bleeding or treat infection.

When a pregnancy goes wrong, it takes away a valuable contributor from the family (sometimes permanently) and places an additional strain on resources and manpower.

Pregnancy Complications

The reasons that women could cease to become productive group members (or even die) during pregnancy or childbirth include the following:

Hyperemesis gravidarum. Simply put, this is excessive vomiting in early pregnancy. Everyone's nauseous when they're pregnant, but a few will have such extreme vomiting as to become severely dehydrated. Without IV fluid replacement, some of these patients might not survive.

Miscarriage. Approximately 10 percent of all pregnancies end in miscarriage. When a woman miscarries, she might not pass all of the dead tissue relating to the pregnancy. This tissue may become infected or cause excessive bleeding.

The treatment in this case would be dilatation and curettage (D&C), a procedure in which scrapers called curettes are used to remove the retained tissue. Without the right equipment and experience, some women might succumb.

Pregnancy-induced hypertension. Blood pressure may rise to dangerous levels and cause alarming amounts of swelling, sometimes throughout the body. This mostly is seen in the last 3 months of a first pregnancy. Left untreated, this condition leads to seizures and can be life threatening. Without modern facilities, bed rest (lying on the left side is best) may be just about all that you can do.

Childbirth issues. The delivery itself, although usually straightforward, can be fraught with complications. Excessive bleeding could occur before, during or after delivery due to vaginal tears or premature separation of the placenta from the uterus. The placenta ordinarily is expelled spontaneously within minutes after the delivery; however, there are occasions where it is "stuck" and must be manually removed. In these cases, portions of the placenta may remain lodged in the uterine walls, leading to bleeding and/or infection. Failure of the uterine walls to contract after delivery may also cause hemorrhage.

Pregnancy Care Basics

You may find yourself responsible for the care of a pregnant woman. It will be important to know how to support that pregnancy and, eventually, deliver that baby.

Without access to prenatal megavitamins, babies will be smaller at birth. This may also not be so bad, since having a Caesarean section won't be available. It's less traumatic for the mother to deliver a 6–7 pound baby than a 10 pounder.

Despite all the possible complications mentioned in the previous section, pregnancy is still a natural process. It usually proceeds without major complications and ends in the delivery of a normal baby. Although your pregnant patient will not be as productive for the survival group as she would ordinarily be, she will probably still be able to contribute to help make your efforts a success. The medic will need to know pregnancy care and how to deliver the fetus.

Today, we have simple tests that can identify pregnancy almost before a woman misses her period, but what if these tests are no longer available? You will have to rely on the following tried and true signs and symptoms to identify the condition:

- ⚕ Absent menstruation
- ⚕ Tender breasts
- ⚕ Nausea and vomiting
- ⚕ Darkening of the nipples, areola, or both
- ⚕ Fatigue
- ⚕ Frequent urination
- ⚕ Backache

These symptoms, in combination, indicate pregnancy. The timing of each will be variable: some will be noticed earlier than others. It should be noted that this investigation will be necessary only in those women experiencing their first pregnancy. Once a woman has been pregnant, she will usually just know when it happens again.

For more about the monitoring and care of a pregnancy, consider getting a copy of our book *The Survival Medicine Handbook*.

Normal Delivery

As the woman approaches her due date, several things will happen. The fetus will begin to drop lower in the pelvis. The patient's abdomen may look different, or the top of the uterus (fundus) may appear lower. As the neck of the uterus (cervix) relaxes, the patient may notice a mucus-like discharge, sometimes with a bloody component. This is referred to as the "bloody show" and is usually a sign that things will be happening soon.

If you examine your patient vaginally by gently inserting two fingers of a gloved hand, you'll notice the cervix is firm, like your nose, when the due date is approaching and soft, like your lips, when it isn't. This softening of the cervix is called "effacement." As labor progresses, the cervical walls will thin out until they are as thin as paper.

Dilation of the cervical opening will be slow at first, and speed up once it reaches about 3–4 cm. At this level of dilation, you will be able to place two (normal-sized) fingertips in the cervix and feel something firm; this is the baby's head. Frequent vaginal exams are invasive, however, and not necessary in most cases.

Contractions will start becoming more frequent. To identify a contraction, feel the skin on the soft area of your cheek, and then touch your forehead. A contraction will feel firm like your forehead. False labor contractions will be irregular and will go away with bed rest (especially when the patient lies on her left side) and hydration. If contractions are coming faster and more furious, even with bed rest and hydration, it is probably the real thing! A gush of watery fluid from the vagina will often signify the "water breaking" (rupture of the amniotic sac) and is also a sign of impending labor and delivery. The timing, however, will be highly variable.

To prepare for delivery, wash your hands and put gloves on. Then, set up clean sheets so that there will be the least contamination possible. Tuck a sheet under the mother's buttocks and spread it on your lap so that the baby, which comes out very slippery, will land onto the sheet instead of landing on the floor if you lose your grip. Place a towel on the mother's belly; this is where the baby will go once it is delivered. Delivery kits are available online with everything you need, including drapes, clamps, and bulb syringes. To prevent infection, avoid touching anything but mother and baby if you can.

As the labor progresses, the baby's head will move down the birth canal and the vagina will begin to bulge. When the baby's head begins to become visible, it is called "crowning." If the water has not yet broken (which can happen even at this late stage), the lining of the bag of water will appear as a slick gray surface. Some pressure on the membrane will rupture it, which is okay at this point. It might help the process along.

To make space, place two gloved fingers along the edge of the vagina by the perineum, the area between the vagina and anus. Using gentle pressure, move your fingers from side to side. This will stretch the area somewhat to give the baby a little more room to come out.

With each contraction, the baby's head will come out a little more. Don't be concerned if it goes back after the contraction. It should make steady progress, with more and more of the head becoming visible. Encourage the mother to help by taking a deep breath with each contraction and then pushing while slowly exhaling.

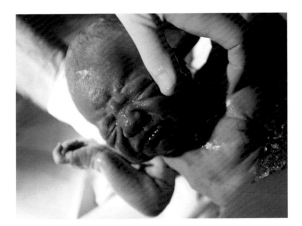

As the baby's head emerges, it will usually face straight down or up, and then turn to the side. The cord might appear to be wrapped around its neck. If this is the case, gently slip the cord over the baby's head. In cases where the cord is very tight and is preventing delivery, you may choose to doubly clamp it and cut between. This will release the tension and make delivery easier.

Next, gently hold each side of the baby's head and apply gentle traction straight down. This will help the top shoulder out of the birth canal. Then, raise the head to release the bottom shoulder. Once the shoulders are out, the baby will deliver with one last push. The mother can now rest.

Put the baby immediately on the mother's belly and clean out its nose and mouth with a bulb syringe. It will usually begin crying, which is a good sign that it is a vigorous infant. If it doesn't, stimulate it by rubbing the baby's back. (Spanking its bottom is more a cliché than recommended procedure.)

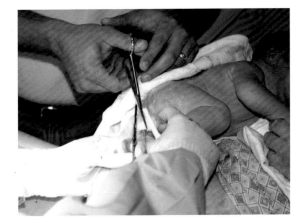

Dry the baby and wrap it up in a small towel or blanket. At this point, you may clamp the cord twice (2 inches apart) with Kelly or umbilical clamps, and cut in between with a scissors. There is no hurry to perform this procedure.

Once the baby has delivered, it's the placenta's turn. Be patient: In most cases, the placenta will deliver by itself in a few minutes. Pulling on the umbilical cord to force the placenta out is usually a bad idea. Breaking the cord because the placenta will not come out will require your placing your hand deep in the uterus to extract it. This is traumatic and can introduce infection. You can ask the mother to give a push when it's clear the placenta is almost out.

If traction is necessary for some reason to get the placenta to deliver, place your fingers above the pubic bone and press as you apply mild traction. This will prevent the uterus' being turned inside out (a potentially life-threatening situation) if the placenta is stubborn. A moderate amount of bleeding is not unusual after delivery of the afterbirth.

Once the placenta is out, examine it. The fetal surface (the surface to which the fetus was attached) is grey and shiny; turn it inside out and you will see the maternal surface, which looks like a rough version of liver. If a portion of the placenta remains inside, you may have to extract it manually.

The uterus (the top of which is now around the level of the belly button) contracts to control bleeding naturally. In a long labor, the uterus may be as tired as the mother after delivery and may be slow to contract. This may cause excessive bleeding. Gentle massage of the top of the fundus will make it firm again and thus limit blood loss. You may have to do this from time to time during the first 24 hours or so after delivery.

Monitor the mother closely for excessive bleeding over the next few days. In normal situations, the bleeding will become more and more watery as time progresses. This is normal. Also keep an eye out for evidence of fever, foul discharge, or other issues.

Place the baby on the mother's breast soon after delivery. This will begin the secretion of colostrum, a form of milk produced by the breast that appears as a thick, yellowish liquid; it is rich in substances that will increase the baby's resistance to infection. Suckling also causes the uterus to contract, a factor in decreasing blood loss.

It should be noted that there are different schools of thought regarding some of the above information about delivery. Remember that your goal is to have an end result of a healthy mother and baby, both physically and emotionally.

IX.

✚ ✚ ✚

MEDICATIONS

ESSENTIAL OVER-THE-COUNTER DRUGS

Over-the-counter (OTC) medications are useful for a wide variety of problems. These drugs are widely available and easy to accumulate in quantity. As such, they are ideal for the survival medic's cache of medical supplies. The *Physicians' Desk Reference* puts out a guide to OTC medications with descriptions, images, risks, benefits, dosages, and side effects. Consider this book for your survival medical library.

There are a dozen meds you absolutely must have in quantity as part of your medical supplies. The medications will be listed by their generic names, with US brand names in parenthesis where applicable. Adult doses are listed. They are described below in no particular order:

Ibuprofen (Motrin, Advil), 200 mg: A popular pain reliever, anti-inflammatory, and fever reducer. This medication is useful for many different problems, which makes it especially useful as a stockpile item. It can alleviate pain from strains, sprains, arthritis, and traumatic injury and help reduce inflammation in the injured area. Ibuprofen is also useful in reducing fevers from infections. The downside to this medication is that it can cause stomach upset. Ibuprofen in this dosage can be used 1–2 every 4 hours, 3 every 6 hours, or 4 every 8 hours.

Acetaminophen (Tylenol), 325 mg: Another popular pain reliever and fever reducer, acetaminophen can be used for all of the problems that you can take ibuprofen for, with the added benefit of not causing stomach irritation or thinning the blood. Unfortunately, it has no significant anti-inflammatory effect. This drug is excellent for treatment of pain and fevers in children at lower doses. Tylenol comes in regular and extra strength (650 mg); adults should take 1–2 every 4 hours.

Aspirin, 325 mg: Aspirin has been around since the late nineteenth century as a pain reliever, fever reducer, and anti-inflammatory. It has blood thinning properties as well, and may be all we have to help those with medical issues that require the use of anticoagulants. It is also useful to treat older folks with coronary artery disease. If you suspect someone of having a heart attack, have them chew an adult aspirin immediately; 1 baby aspirin (81 mg) daily may help prevent coronary artery disease. Have patients take 2 adult aspirin every 4 hours for pain, fever, and inflammation.

Loperamide (Imodium), 2 mg: Food and water are highly likely to have contamination issues in off-grid situations, so this medication is essential as an antidiarrheal. By slowing intestinal motility, less water loss will occur from the body. This decreases the chance of developing dehydration, a known killer in austere settings. With diarrheal disease, you often have nausea and vomiting, so you will also want to have:

Meclizine (Antivert), 12.5, 25, 50 mg: Meclizine is a medication that helps prevent nausea and vomiting. Often used to prevent motion sickness, meclizine also helps with dizziness and tends to act as a sedative. As such, it may have uses as a sleep aid or antianxiety medication. To prevent motion sickness, patients should take 1 tablet (25 mg) 1 hour before traveling for dizziness, anxiety, or to induce sleep, 50–100, divided into several doses, should be taken daily.

Antibiotic ointment (Neosporin, bacitracin, Bactroban): When injuries break the skin, it puts us in danger of infections that could lead to a life-threatening condition. Antibiotic ointment is applied at the site of injury to prevent infections. It should be noted that antibiotic ointment won't cure a deep infection; you would need oral or IV antibiotics for that, but using the ointment immediately after an injury will give you a good chance at preventing it. Apply 3–4 times a day.

Diphenhydramine (Benadryl), 25 mg, 50 mg: Diphenhydramine is an antihistamine that alleviates the itching, rashes, nasal congestion, and other symptoms of allergic reactions. It also helps drain the nasal passages in some respiratory infections. At the higher 50 mg dose, it makes an effective sleep aid. The recommended dose is 25 mg every 6 hours for mild reactions; 50 mg every 6 hours for severe reactions, anxiety, or sleep. Diphenhydramine also comes in an ointment for skin eruptions.

Pseudoephedrine (Sudafed): Pseudoephedrine is a nasal decongestant for respiratory infections like the common cold or influenza. Obtain small amounts at a time, as it is also an ingredient in the manufacture of the recreational drug methamphetamine, and purchases may be monitored.

Hydrocortisone cream (1 percent): Highly useful for rashes, this cream is used for various types of dermatitis that causes redness, flakiness, itching, and thickening of the skin. It's a mild steroid that reduces inflammation and, as such, the various symptoms of allergic dermatitis, eczema, diaper rash, etc. Apply 3–4 times a day to affected area.

Omeprazole (Prilosec), 20–40mg; cimetidine (Tagamet), 200–800mg; ranitidine (Zantac), 75–150 mg: In a situation where we may be eating things we're not accustomed to, we may have issues with stomach acid. The above antacids will calm heartburn, queasiness, and stomach upset. Calcium carbonate (Tums) or magnesium sulfate (Maalox) is also fine in solid form. These medications are also useful for acid reflux and ulcer disease.

Clotrimazole, miconazole cream or powder (Lotrimin™, Monistat): Infections can be bacterial, but they can also be caused by fungus. Common examples of this are athlete's foot, vaginal yeast infections, ringworm, and jock itch. These conditions will be just as common in times of trouble as they are now, if not more. Apply clotrimazole 2 times a day externally or miconazole 1 time a day intravaginally.

Multivitamins: In a societal collapse, the unavailability of a good variety of food may lead to dietary deficiencies, not just in calories but in vitamins and minerals. Vitamin C deficiency, for example, leads to scurvy. To prevent these issues, you should have plenty of multivitamins, commercial or natural, in your medical storage. You won't necessarily have to take these on a daily basis; many multivitamins give you more than you need if taken daily.

The good news is that you can probably obtain a significant amount of all of the above drugs for a reasonable amount of money. To retain full potency, these medications should be obtained in pill or capsule form; avoid the liquid versions if possible. Remember that medications should be stored in cool, dry, dark places.

PAIN MEDICATIONS

It stands to reason that minor issues with discomfort now will be multiplied by the increased workload demands of a power-down situation. Sprains, strains, and worse will be part and parcel of any long-term survival situation. Therefore, any person who hasn't considered providing for pain issues in times of trouble is not medically prepared. It's a good idea to have a working knowledge of the actions and uses of various pain medications.

As pain is variable, there are many different types of drugs available that have different mechanisms of action for pain relief (analgesia), as described below.

Nonsteroidal anti-inflammatories (NSAIDS): These drugs act to decrease inflammation and fever as well as pain. The most popular NSAIDs are ibuprofen and aspirin; naproxen is another NSAID that is available without a prescription. For quick relief from pain, the shorter-acting ibuprofen or aspirin is superior to naproxen. Naproxen may not have an effect until a couple of doses, but works well for long-term relief.

Acetaminophen: This drug relieves pain by changing the body's sensitivity to things that cause pain (its pain threshold), and also lowers fever. This drug is often as effective as NSAIDs for pain and has fewer side effects (unless you have liver disease). Acetaminophen has no anti-inflammatory action, however; therefore, it may be less effective than NSAIDs for some conditions.

Steroids: Corticosteroids exert their effect upon pain by a very strong anti-inflammatory action. The most common steroids used for inflammation are prednisone and cortisone. They can be taken orally or are sometimes injected directly into damaged and inflamed joints. Long-term use of steroids is associated with a whole gamut of side effects and must be used with the utmost caution.

Muscle relaxants: These drugs not only relax injured muscles but also have a sedative effect. A common one is cyclobenzaprine (Flexeril). These are especially helpful for back strains or other injuries that cause muscle spasms.

Opioids: Narcotics are used for pain in severe cases and act by modifying pain-signal transmission in the brain. If you have had surgery, you likely have been given these medications for pain relief during recovery.

Antianxiety and antidepressant agents: Drugs such as Xanax or Prozac may have an effect on pain by relieving psychogenic factors, such as anxiety or depression; this enables the patient to better deal with their pain issues. They work by adjusting the level of certain chemicals in the brain tissue.

Antiseizure medication: Some anticonvulsant drugs, such as Tegretol, used for epilepsy are useful to calm damaged nerves and are possible options for neuropathic pain.

Combination drugs: Some pain medications are combinations of different drugs. Percocet, for example, is acetaminophen and oxycodone (an opioid). Some are used alternatively during the day, for example, an NSAID may be prescribed between doses of an opioid.

Most of these drugs are by prescription only, and it will be unlikely that you'll be able to stockpile large quantities of any but the nonprescription versions. As such, it will be important to know about some natural alternatives you have for pain relief.

NATURAL PAIN RELIEF

In a long-term survival situation, your limited supplies of the medicines described above will eventually run out. This leaves you with natural alternatives from products that you can grow yourself or, perhaps, find in your environment. Their benefit will vary from person to person. We describe some of these alternatives below.

Capsaicin: This is an ingredient in chili peppers that decreases pain sensation by deactivating pain receptors. This is especially helpful for those who suffer from headache, muscle ache, and arthritis and those with neuropathic pain. The most pain relief occurs after using capsaicin for a month or so.

Salicin: The original ingredient in the first pharmaceutical, aspirin, salicin has been manufactured since the nineteenth century. Salicin is found in the bark of willow, aspen, and poplar trees. Pain sufferers can get relief by chewing on strips of the green underbark (not outer bark) of these trees or making a tea out of it. Like aspirin, salicin will also help reduce fever.

Arnica: A natural anti-inflammatory, this substance reduces swelling and, therefore, discomfort from injuries to joints and muscles.

Methylsulfonyl-methane (MSM): Derived from sulfur, this substance helps slow down degeneration from joint disease, especially when combined with glucosamine and chondroitin. Over the course of time, arthritis sufferers often report significant pain relief.

Curcumin: The herb turmeric contains this substance, which increases the body's defense against inflammation, thereby decreasing pain.

Ginger root: A tea made of ginger root is thought to decrease inflammation and provide relief from stomach pain.

Boswellia: This herb from India produces certain acidic compounds that are touted as useful for chronic pain and is said to decrease inflammation.

S-adenosylmethionine (SAM-e): SAM-e seems to reduce inflammation and increase neurotransmitters in the brain that increase the sensation of well-being. Taking this supplement long-term seems to give the best likelihood of obtaining pain relief.

Be open to every strategy available to deal with a medical issue; there are a lot of tools in the medical woodshed, and you should take advantage of all methods that may keep your family and community healthy in uncertain times.

STOCKPILING MEDICATIONS

Accumulating medications for a possible collapse may be simple when it comes to getting ibuprofen and other nonprescription drugs. It will be a major issue, however, for those who need to stockpile prescription medicines; most people don't have a relationship with a physician who can or will accommodate their requests. Antibiotics are one example of medications that will be very useful in a collapse situation. Obtaining these drugs in quantity will be difficult, to say the least.

The inability to store antibiotic supplies is going to cost some poorly prepared individuals their lives in a collapse situation. Incidence of infection will be much larger when people have to fend for themselves and are injured as a result. Any strenuous activities performed in a power-down situation, especially ones that most of us aren't accustomed to, will cause various cuts and scratches. These wounds will very likely be dirty. Within a relatively short time, dirty wounds can become infected, appearing red, swollen, and warm to the touch.

Treatment of such infections at an early stage improves the chance that they will heal quickly and perhaps avoid unnecessary complications, even death. The availability of antibiotics would make it possible to deal with the issue safely and effectively.

The following advice, on antibiotic options, is contrary to standard medical practice, and is a strategy that is appropriate only in the event of societal collapse. If there are modern medical resources available to you, seek them out.

Antibiotic Options

We have kept parrots for many years. Currently, we are growing tilapia as a food fish in an aquaculture pond. After years of using aquatic medicines on fish and avian medicines on birds, we decided to evaluate these drugs for their potential use in collapse situations. They seemed to be good candidates: All were widely available, available in different varieties, and didn't require a medical license to obtain them.

A close inspection of the bottles revealed that, often, the only ingredient was the drug itself, identical to those obtained by prescription at the local pharmacy. If the bottle says Fish Mox, for example, the sole ingredient is amoxicillin, which is an antibiotic commonly used in humans.

A number of these aquatic and avian antibiotics come only in dosages that correspond to pediatric or adult human dosages. Why should this be? Why should a 1-inch-long guppy require the same dosage of, say, Amoxicillin (aquatic version: Fish Mox Forte) as a 180-pound adult human? I was told that it was because of the dilution of the drug in water. However, at the time of this writing, there are few instructions that tell you how much to put in a ½-gallon fishbowl as opposed to a 200-gallon aquarium.

Finally, my acid test was to look at the pills or capsules themselves. The aquatic or avian drug had to be identical to that found in bottles of the corresponding human medicine. When I opened a bottle of Fish Mox Forte and compared it with a bottle of human amoxicillin 500 mg produced by Dava Pharmaceuticals, I found they were the same: red and pink capsules, with the letters and numbers WC 731 on them.

Logically, then, it makes sense to believe that they are manufactured in the same way that human antibiotics are. Further, it is my opinion that they are probably from the same batches; some go to human pharmacies, and some go to veterinary pharmacies.

This is not to imply that all antibiotic medications sold for animals meet my criteria. Many cat, dog, and livestock antibiotics contain additives that might even cause ill effects on a human being. Look only for those veterinary drugs that have the antibiotic as the *sole* ingredient.

Here is a list of the products that meet my criteria and that I believe will be beneficial to have as supplies and are discussed in the next section:

- Fish Mox (amoxicillin 250 mg)
- Fish Mox Forte (amoxicillin 500 mg)
- Fish Cillin (ampicillin 250 mg)
- Fish Flex (Keflex 250 mg)
- Fish Flex Forte (Keflex 500 mg)
- Fish Zole (metronidazole 250 mg)
- Fish Pen (penicillin 250 mg)
- Fish Pen Forte (penicillin 500 mg)
- Fish Cycline (tetracycline 250 mg)
- Fish Flox (ciprofloxacin 250 mg)
- Fish Cin (clindamycin 150 mg)

- Bird Biotic (doxycycline 100 mg). Used in birds, but the antibiotic is, again, the sole ingredient.
- Bird Sulfa (Sulfamethoxazole 400 mg/Trimethoprin 80 mg). Also used for birds.

These medications are available without a prescription from many online sites. They come in lots of 30–100 tablets, and it appears that you could get as much as you need to stockpile for survival purposes. These quantities would be close to impossible to obtain even from the most sympathetic physician.

Of course, anyone could be allergic to one or another of these antibiotics, but it would be a very rare individual who would be allergic to all of them. There is a 10 percent chance for cross-reactivity between penicillin drugs and Keflex. (If you are allergic to penicillin, you could also be allergic to Keflex.) For penicillin-allergic people, there are safe alternatives that are suitable. Any of the following antibiotics should not cause a reaction in a patient allergic to penicillin-family drugs:

- Doxycycline
- Metronidazole
- Tetracycline
- Ciprofloxacin
- Clindamycin
- Sulfa drugs

I have personally used some (not all) of these antibiotics on myself without any ill effects. Whenever I have used them, they have been indistinguishable from human antibiotics in their effects.

Having said this, I *do not* recommend self-treatment in any circumstance that does not involve the complete long-term loss of access to modern medical care. This is a strategy to save lives in a postcalamity scenario only.

Antibiotics are used at different doses for different illnesses. It's important to have as much information as possible on medications that you plan to store, so consider purchasing a hard copy of the latest *Physicians' Desk Reference*. This book has just about every bit of information that exists on a particular drug.

Under each medicine, you will find the "indications," which are the medical conditions that the drug is used for. Also listed will be the dosages, risks, side effects, and even how the medicine works in the body. It's okay to get last year's book; the information doesn't change a great deal from one year to the next.

Antibiotic Overuse

It's important to understand that you will not want to indiscriminately use antibiotics for every minor ailment that comes along. In a collapse, the medic is also a quartermaster of sorts; you will want to wisely dispense that limited and, yes, precious supply of lifesaving drugs. You must walk a fine line between observant patient management (doing nothing) and aggressive management (doing everything). Liberal use of antibiotics is a poor strategy for a few reasons:

Overuse can foster the spread of resistant bacteria, as you'll remember from the salmonellosis (food poisoning caused by the bacteria in the *Salmonella* genus) outbreak in turkeys in 2011. Millions of pounds of turkey meat were discarded after 100 people were sent to the hospital with severe diarrheal disease.

- Potential allergic reactions may occur that could lead to anaphylactic shock.
- Making a diagnosis may be more difficult. If you give antibiotics *before* you're sure what medical problem you're actually dealing with, you might "mask" the condition. In other words, symptoms could be temporarily improved that would have helped you know what disease your patient has. This could cost you valuable time in determining the correct treatment.

You can see that judicious use of antibiotics, under your close supervision, is necessary to fully utilize their benefits. Discourage your group members from using these drugs without first consulting you.

How to Use Antibiotics

There are many antibiotics, but which that are accessible to the average person would be good additions to your medical storage? When do you use a particular drug? In this section, we discuss antibiotics (all available in veterinary form without a prescription) that you will want in your medical arsenal:

- Amoxicillin 250 mg or 500 mg (Fish Mox, Fish Mox Forte)
- Ciprofloxacin 250 mg or 500 mg (Fish Flox, Fish Flox Forte)
- Cephalexin 250 mg or 500 mg (Fish Flex, Fish Flex Forte)
- Metronidazole 250 mg (Fish Zole)
- Doxycycline 100 mg (Bird Biotic)
- Ampicillin 250 mg or 500 mg (Fish Cillin, Fish Cillin Forte)
- Sulfamethoxazole 400 mg/Trimethoprim 80 mg (Bird Sulfa)
- Clindamycin 150 mg (Fish Cin)
- Azithromycin 250 mg (Aquatic Azithromycin)

There are various others that you can choose, but these selections will give you the opportunity to treat many illnesses and have enough variety so that even those with penicillin allergies will have options.

Other than allergies, there are other times when a particular antibiotic (or other drug) should not be used. Many medications, for example, are not recommended for use during pregnancy. Sometimes, this is because lab studies have shown birth defects in animal fetuses exposed to the drug. Other times, it is because no studies on pregnant women or animals have yet been performed.

There are additional circumstances where a particular medication should not be used. There may be warnings about mixing one drug with another because there may be a dangerous interaction between them. For example, taking the antibiotic metronidazole (Fish Zole) and drinking alcohol will make you vomit. Some drug interactions may cause the effect of one of them to become stronger or weaker. A certain medicine, for example, may decrease the effect of another when taken together. You also may wish to avoid some drugs because of their side effects. This information is freely available; you just have to spend some time absorbing it.

Different physicians may use a specific antibiotic for different purposes and to treat a variety of infections. Some will not agree with everything you see written in this book. Below are examples of how to use some antibiotics.

Amoxicillin

Amoxicillin (veterinary equivalent: Fish Mox, Fish Mox Forte, Aqua Mox): comes in 250 mg and 500 mg doses, usually taken 3 times a day. Amoxicillin is the most popular antibiotic prescribed to children, usually in liquid form. It is more versatile and better absorbed and tolerated than the older pencillins and is acceptable for use during pregnancy. Ampicillin (Fish Cillin) and cephalexin (Fish Flex) are related drugs. Amoxicillin may be used for the following diseases:

- Anthrax (prevention or treatment of cutaneous transmission)
- Chlamydia infection (sexually transmitted)
- Urinary tract infection (bladder and kidney infections)
- *Helicobacter pylori* infection (causes peptic ulcer)
- Lyme disease (transmitted by ticks)
- Otitis media (middle-ear infection)
- Pneumonia (lung infection)
- Sinusitis
- Skin or soft tissue infection (cellulitis, boils)
- Actinomycosis (causes abscesses in humans and livestock)
- Bronchitis
- Tonsillitis and pharyngitis (strep throat)

You can see that amoxicillin is a versatile drug. It is even safe for use during pregnancy, but all of the above is a lot of information. How do you determine what dose and frequency would be appropriate for which individual? Let's take an example: Otitis media is a common ear infection often seen in children. Amoxicillin is often the drug of choice for this condition. That is, it is recommended to be used *first* when you make a diagnosis of otitis media. The drug of choice for a particular ailment can change over time on the basis of new scientific evidence.

Before administering this medication, however, you would want to determine that your patient is not allergic to amoxicillin. The most common form of allergy would appear as a rash, but diarrhea, itchiness, and even respiratory difficulty could also manifest. If you see any of these symptoms, you should discontinue your treatment and look for other options. Antibiotics such as azithromycin or sulfamethoxazole/trimethoprim (Bird Sulfa) could be a second-line solution in this case.

Once you have identified amoxicillin as your treatment of choice to treat your patient's ear infection, you will want to determine the dosage. As otitis media often occurs in children, you might have to break a tablet in half or open the capsule to separate out a portion that would be appropriate. For amoxicillin, you would give 20–50 mg per kilogram (2.2 pounds) of body weight (20–30 mg per kilogram for infants younger than 4 months old). This would be useful if you have to give the drug to a toddler who is less than 30 pounds.

A common older child's dosage would be 250 mg, and a common maximum dosage for adults would be 500 mg 3 times a day. Luckily (or by design), these dosages are exactly how the commercially made aquatic medications come in the bottle. Take this dosage orally 3 times a day for 10–14 days (2 times a day for infants). All of the above information can be found in the *Physicians' Desk Reference*.

If your child is too small to swallow a pill whole, you could make a mixture with water (a suspension). To make a liquid suspension, crush a tablet or empty a capsule into a small glass of water and drink it; then, fill the glass again and drink that (particles may adhere to the walls of the glass). You can add some flavoring to make it taste better.

Do not chew or make a liquid out of time-released capsules of any medication; you will wind up losing some of the gradual release effect and perhaps get too much into your system at once. These medications should be plainly marked "time-released."

You will probably see improvement within 3 days, but don't be tempted to stop the antibiotic therapy until you're done with the entire 10–14 days. Sometimes you'll kill most of the bacteria, but some colonies may persist and multiply if you prematurely end the treatment. This is often cited as a cause of antibiotic resistance. In a long-term survival situation, however, you might be down to your last few pills and have to make some tough decisions.

Ciprofloxacin

A useful antibiotic option is ciprofloxacin (veterinary equivalent: Fish Flox). Ciprofloxacin is in the fluoroquinolone family. It kills bacteria by inhibiting the reproduction of DNA and bacterial proteins. This drug usually comes in 250 mg and 500 mg doses.

Ciprofloxacin (Cipro) can be used for the following conditions:

- Bladder or other urinary infections, especially in females
- Prostate infections
- Some types of lower respiratory infections, such as pneumonia
- Acute sinusitis
- Skin infections (such as cellulitis)
- Bone and joint infections
- Infectious diarrhea
- Typhoid fever caused by *Salmonella*
- Inhalational anthrax

In most cases, you should give 500 mg 2 times a day for 7–14 days, with the exception of bone and joint infections (4–6 weeks) and anthrax (60 days). You can get away with 250 mg doses for 3 days for most mild urinary infections. Generally, you would want to continue the medication for 2 days after improvement is noted.

Unlike amoxicillin, many antibiotics may not be safe for use in certain situations. For example, ciprofloxacin has not been approved for use during pregnancy. Among its side effects, Cipro has been reported to cause weakness occasionally in muscles and tendons. It may also cause joint and muscle complications in children, so it is restricted in pediatric use to urinary tract infections and pyelonephritis due to *E. coli* (the most common type) and occasionally to inhalational anthrax.

In children, the dosage is measured by multiplying 10 mg by the weight of the child, in kilograms (1 kg equals 2.2 pounds). The maximum dose should not exceed 400 mg total twice a day, even if the child weighs more than 100 pounds. Ciprofloxacin should be taken with 8 ounces of water.

Cephalexin

Cephalexin (veterinary equivalent: Fish Flex, Fish Flex Forte) is an antibiotic in the cephalosporin family. It is different from but cross-reactive with the penicillin family; this means that a percentage of penicillin-allergic patients will also be allergic to cephalosporins.

Cephalexin works by interfering with the bacteria's cell wall formation. This causes the defective wall to rupture, killing the bacteria. This antibiotic is useful treating the following:

- Cystitis (bladder infections)
- Otitis media (ear infections)
- Pharyngitis (sore throats)
- Skin or soft-tissue infection (infected cuts)
- Osteomyelitis (infections of the bone)
- Prostatitis (prostate infections)
- Pyelonephritis (kidney infections)
- Upper respiratory tract infection

Cephalexin is also used as a preventative before surgical procedures in people who are at risk for heart-valve infections. It is also one of the few antibiotics that is thought to be safe to use during pregnancy. Cephalexin is marketed in the United States under the name Keflex.

To use this medication, you would normally give 250 mg (Fish Flex) or 500mg (Fish Flex Forte) every 6 hours for 7–14 days. Severe bacterial infections may require an additional week of treatment. Infections of the bone (osteomyelitis) are particularly dangerous and require 4–6 weeks of therapy.

Pediatric dosages are calculated using 12.5–25 mg per kilogram of body weight orally every 6–12 hours. (Don't exceed adult dosages.)

Doxycycline

Another useful antibiotic in a collapse would be doxycycline (veterinary equivalent: Bird Biotic). Doxycycline is a member of the tetracycline family and is also acceptable to use with patients who are allergic to penicillin. It inhibits the production of bacterial protein, which prevents its reproduction. Doxycycline is marketed under various names, including Vibramycin and Vibra-Tabs.

Doxycycline is an extraordinarily versatile drug. Indications for its usage include the following:

- *E. coli*, *Shigella,* and *Enterobacter* infections (diarrheal disease)
- Chlamydia (sexually transmitted disease)
- Lyme disease
- Rocky Mountain spotted fever
- Anthrax
- Cholera
- Plague

- Gum disease (severe gingivitis, periodontitis)
- Folliculitis (boils)
- Acne and other inflammatory skin diseases, such as hidradenitis (seen in armpits and groins)
- Some lower respiratory tract (pneumonia) and urinary tract infections
- Upper respiratory infections caused by strep
- Methicillin-resistant *Staphylococcus aureus* (MRSA) infections
- Malaria (prevention)
- Some parasitic worm infections (kills bacteria in their gut that they need to survive)

In the case of Rocky Mountain spotted fever, doxycycline is indicated even for use in children. Otherwise, doxycycline is not meant for those younger than 8 years old. It has not been approved for use during pregnancy.

The recommended doxycycline dosage for most types of bacterial infections in adults is 100 mg–200 mg per day for 7–14 days. For chronic (long-term) or more serious infections, treatment can be carried out for a longer time. Children should receive 1–2 mg per pound of body weight per day. For anthrax, the treatment should be prolonged to 60 days. As prevention against malaria, adults should use 100 mg per day.

Although antibiotics may be helpful in diarrheal disease, always start with hydration and symptomatic relief. Prolonged diarrhea, high fevers, and bleeding are reasons to consider antibiotic use. The risk is that one of the most common side effects of antibiotics is . . . diarrhea!

Azithromycin

Another antibiotic available in an aquatic equivalent is azithromycin 250 mg. Azithromycin is a member of the macrolide (erythromycin) family and can be found also as Aquatic Azithromycin. It works by stopping the growth and multiplication of bacteria. I prefer it to aquatic erythromycin powder (Fish Mycin), as azithromycin is available in a capsule and thus more easily administered.

Azithromycin can be used to treat various types of the following:

- Bronchitis
- Pneumonia

- Ear infections
- Skin infections
- Throat infections (some)
- Sinusitis
- Tonsillitis
- Typhoid fever
- Gonorrhea
- Chlamydia
- Whooping cough
- Lyme disease (early stages)

Azithromycin is taken 250 mg or 500 mg 1 time a day for a relatively short course of treatment (usually 5 days). The first dose is often a "double dose," twice as much as the remainder of the doses given. This method of taking the drug is known in the United States as a Z-Pack.

For acute bacterial sinusitis, azithromycin may be taken 1 time a day for 3 days. If you are taking the 500 mg dosage and have side effects, such as nausea and vomiting, diarrhea, or dizziness, drop down to the lower dosage. Azithromycin is not known to cause problems in pregnant patients.

Clindamycin

Clindamycin (Fish Cin) is part of the lincomycin antibiotic family of drugs. It, like azithromycin, works by slowing or stopping the growth of bacteria. It works best on bacteria that are anaerobic, which means that they thrive in the absence of oxygen. It can be used to treat the following:

- Acne
- Dental infections
- Soft-tissue (skin, etc.) infections
- Peritonitis (inflammation of the peritoneum, which lines the inner wall of the abdomen and covers most of the abdominal organs)
- Pneumonia and lung abscesses
- Uterine infections (such as after miscarriage or childbirth)
- Blood infections
- Pelvic infections
- MRSA (methicillin-resistant *Staphylococcus aureus* infections)

- Parasitic infections (malaria, toxoplasmosis)
- Anthrax

Clindamycin is given in 150 mg or 300 mg doses every 6 hours with a glass of water. It should be used with caution in individuals with a history of gastrointestinal disease, as it can cause diarrhea during treatment. Sometimes, a very serious colitis (infection of the intestine) can develop. This drug is, like azithromycin, pregnancy category B, which means that no ill effects have been determined in animal studies. With most drugs, testing cannot be done ethically on pregnant humans, so very few drugs are willing to say that any medicine is completely safe during pregnancy.

Ciprofloxacin, clindamycin, doxycycline, and azithromycin are acceptable for use in patients with Penicillin allergies. This is not to say that you might not have a different allergy to one or the other, however.

Metronidazole

Metronidazole (aquatic equivalent: Fish Zole) 250 mg is an antibiotic in the nitroimidazole family that is used primarily to treat infections caused by anaerobic bacteria and protozoa.

Anaerobes are bacteria that do not depend on oxygen to live. Protozoa have been defined as single-cell organisms with animal-like behavior. Many can propel themselves from place to place by the means of a flagellum; a tail-like hair they whip around that enables them to move.

Metronidazole works by blocking some of the functions within bacteria and protozoa, thus resulting in their death. It is better known by the US brand name Flagyl™ and usually comes in 250 mg and 500 mg tablets. Metronidazole is used in the treatment of the following bacterial diseases:

- Diverticulitis (intestinal infection seen in older individuals)
- Peritonitis (infection of the peritoneum, which lines the inner wall of the abdomen and covers most of the abdominal organs)
- Some pneumonias
- Diabetic foot-ulcer infections
- Meningitis (infection of the spinal cord and brain lining)
- Bone and joint infections

- Colitis due to *Clostridia* bacterial species (sometimes caused by taking clindamycin!)
- Endocarditis (heart infection)
- Bacterial vaginosis (common vaginal infection)
- Pelvic inflammatory disease (infection in women that can lead to abscesses)—used in combination with other antibiotics
- Uterine infections (especially after childbirth and miscarriage)
- Dental infections (sometimes in combination with amoxicillin)
- *Helicobacter pylori* infections (causes peptic ulcers)
- Some skin infections

And the following protozoal infections:

- Amoebiasis—dysentery caused by *Entamoeba* species (contaminated water or food)
- Giardiasis—infection of the small intestine caused by *Giardia* species (contaminated water or food)
- Trichomoniasis—vaginal infection caused by a parasite that can be sexually transmitted

Amoebiasis and giardiasis can be caught from drinking what appears to be the purest mountain stream water. Never fail to sterilize all water, regardless of source, before drinking it.

Metronidazole is used in different dosages to treat different illnesses. The following are the dosages and frequency of administration for several:

- **Amoebic dysentery**—750 mg orally 3 times daily for 5–10 days. For children, give 35–50 mg per kilograms of the child's weight per day orally in 3 divided doses for 10 days (no more than adult dosage, of course, regardless of weight).
- **Anaerobic infections (various)**—7.5 mg/kg orally every 6 hours, not to exceed 4 grams daily.
- **Clostridia infections**—250–500 mg orally 4 times daily or 500–750 orally 3 times daily.
- **Giardia**—250 mg orally 3 times daily for 5 days. For children give 15 mg/kg/day orally in 3 divided doses (no more than adult dosage regardless of weight).

- *Helicobacter pylori* (**ulcer disease**)—500–750mg 2 times a day for several days in combination with other drugs, such as Prilosec (omeprazole).
- **Pelvic inflammatory disease (PID)**—500 mg orally 2 times a day for 14 days in combination with other drugs, perhaps doxycycline or azithromycin.
- **Bacterial vaginosis**—500 mg 2 times a day for 7 days.
- **Vaginal trichomoniasis**—2 g single dose (4 500 mg tablets at once) or 1 g twice total.

Like all antibiotics, metronidazole has side effects that you can review by picking up a *Physicians' Desk Reference* or going to drugs.com or rxlist.com. One particular side effect has to do with alcohol: drinking alcohol while on metronidazole will very likely make you vomit. Metronidazole should not be used in pregnancy but can be used in those allergic to penicillin.

Sulfa Drugs

Sulfamethoxazole 400 mg combined with trimethoprim 80 mg (veterinary equivalent: Bird Sulfa) is a combination of medications in the sulfonamide family. This drug is well known as its US brand names Bactrim and Septra. Our British friends may recognize it by the name co-trimoxazole.

Sulfamethoxazole acts as an inhibitor of an important bacterial enzyme. Trimethoprim interferes with the production of folic acid in bacteria, which is necessary to produce DNA. The two antibiotics together are stronger in their effect than alone (at least in laboratory studies).

Sulfamethoxazole 400 mg/trimethoprim 80 mg is effective in the treatment of the following:

- Some upper and lower respiratory infections (chronic bronchitis and pneumonia)
- Kidney and bladder infections
- Ear infections
- Intestinal infections caused by *E. coli* and *Shigella* bacteria
- Skin and wound infections
- Traveler's diarrhea
- Acne

The usual dosage is 1 tablet twice a day for most of the above conditions in adults for 10 days (less in traveler's diarrhea).

The recommended dose for pediatric patients with urinary tract infections or acute otitis media is 8 mg/kg trimethoprim and 40 mg/kg sulfamethoxazole per 24 hours, given in 2 divided doses every 12 hours for 10 days. (Remember that 1 kilogram equals 2.2 pounds.) This medication is contraindicated in infants 2 months old or younger.

In rat studies, the use of this drug was seen to cause birth defects; therefore, it is not used during pregnancy. Sulfamethoxazole 400 mg/trimethoprim 80 mg is well known to cause allergic reactions in some individuals. These reactions are almost as common as seen in penicillin allergies.

Ampicillin

Ampicillin (veterinary equivalent: Fish Cillin) is a member of the penicillin family. It interferes with the ability of bacteria to make cell walls. Ampicillin can be used to treat a number of infections:

- Respiratory-tract infections (bacterial bronchitis)
- Throat infections
- Ear infections
- Cellulitis
- Meningitis
- Urinary tract infections
- Typhoid fever (caused by *Salmonella*)
- Dysentery (caused by *Shigella*)

Ampicillin is usually given to adults in doses of 500 mg 4 times a day for 7–10 days. A common pediatric dosage formula is 6.25–12.5 mg/kg every 6 hours (maximum 2 to 3 g daily). Ampicillin is acceptable for use during pregnancy. Like most antibiotics, it has a stronger effect in intravenous form and can be used intravenously in some cases of septicemia (blood infection) and endocarditis (heart infection).

Antifungal Drugs

Not every medication you use to treat infection will kill bacteria. Viruses and fungi can also cause infection, and you will have to stockpile these drugs as well. Common fungal infections, such as ringworm, athlete's foot, and jock itch will be rampant in wet climates or in situations where you might not be able to change socks or underwear often.

Therefore, it makes sense to keep some antifungal medication around as well. Clotrimazole (Lotrimin) is a good choice here, as it comes in cream or powder and doesn't require a prescription. Medications such as miconazole (Monistat) would be useful for vaginal yeast infections. There is an oral tablet as well, fluconazole (Diflucan), which may be more convenient than creams or powders but requires a prescription.

Antiviral Drugs

Finally, antiviral medications will be useful as well. Many of the infections, especially respiratory, that we assume to be bacterial in nature are more likely to be viral. Antibiotics have no significant effect on viruses; despite this, many patients will demand an antibiotic prescription from their doctors. This overuse is one of the reasons that antibiotic resistance is growing.

One of the most popular antiviral influenza drugs is Tamiflu (oseltamivir). Tamiflu gives effective relief against symptoms of influenza. It can be taken upon exposure to the infection, even before symptoms have begun. If the drug is taken early enough, it might even prevent the illness altogether. Taken in the first 48 hours of a flu-like syndrome, it may decrease the severity and duration of symptoms.

The adult preventative dose of Tamiflu is 75 mg 1 time a day for 10 days. To treat symptoms, take 75 mg 2 times a day for 5 days. For children, use this regimen but with the following doses:

- 15 kg (33 lbs) or less—30 mg dosage
- 16–23 kg (34–51 lbs)—45 mg dosage
- 24–40 kg (52–88 lbs)—60 mg dosage
- More than 40 kg (89 lbs or more)—adult dosage

Tamiflu will not have much effect if taken after the first 48 hours of flu symptoms. Also, it is not proven to be effective against anything other than influenzas (it will not treat Ebola, for example). Despite this, it is wise to obtain prescriptions for every member of your family at the beginning of every flu season.

Other antiviral drugs, such as acyclovir or famcyclovir are usually used to treat conditions related to the herpes virus, such as those listed below.

Shingles (painful skin eruption)
Adults: 800 mg every 4 hours for 5 to 10 days

Children under 40 kg (and older than 2 years): 20 mg/kg 4 times a day for 5 days.

Varicella (chickenpox)
Adults: 800 mg 4 times a day for 5 days
Children under 40 kg (and older than 2 years): 20 mg/kg orally 4 times a day for 5 days.

Oral or genital herpes (herpes simplex)
Adults: 200 mg every 4 hours for 10 days *or* 400 mg 3 times a day for 7–10 days.
Children under 40 kg (and older than 2 years): 40 to 80 mg/kg a day in 3 to 4 divided doses for 5–10 days (maximum dose: 1 g per day).

Don't forget that natural products, such as garlic and honey, have significant properties against certain infections. Garlic, for example, is thought to have antibacterial, antifungal, and antiviral effects. Many people report significant antibacterial and antiviral effect with colloidal silver as well. Before there were antibiotics, there was silver; it is still used in topical creams to prevent infection.

Expiration Dates

A question that we are asked quite often is "What happens when all these drugs I stockpiled pass their expiration date?" The short answer is "In most cases, not very much."

Since 1979, pharmaceutical companies have been required to place expiration dates on their medications. But what do they signify? Officially, the expiration date is the last day that the company will certify that their drug is fully potent. Some believe this means that the medicine in question is useless or in some way dangerous after that date.

This is a false assumption in the vast majority of medicines that come in pill or capsule form. Expiration dates pertain to the strength of the medication in question. You will not grow a third eye in the middle of your forehead simply because the drug has "expired"; it just loses potency.

An exception to this was thought to be tetracycline. A report of kidney damage after taking expired tetracycline was published in the *Journal of the American Medical Association* in 1963. Since that time, the formulation for the drug has changed, and there are few, if any, recent reports of complications. Having said that, I recommend stockpiling doxycycline over tetracycline, as it is a newer-generation drug and might have less resistance issues.

About twenty-five years ago, the US military commissioned a study regarding expiration dates. They had more than a billion dollars' worth of medications stockpiled and were faced with the challenge of destroying huge quantities every two years or so.

The results revealed that 90 percent of medications tested were acceptable for use 8–15 years after the expiration date. The exceptions were mostly in liquid form (insulin, among others). These lose their potency very soon after the date on the package. One sign of this is a change in the color of the liquid, but this is not proof one way or another.

More recently, a program, the Shelf Life Extension Plan (SLEP), evaluated a number of medications stockpiled by the Federal Emergency Management Agency (FEMA); these were mostly antibiotics that had been stockpiled for use in natural disasters that had passed their expiration dates. They also found that the grand majority of medications in pill or capsule form were still good 2–10 years after their expiration dates. The conclusion of the study, published in 2006, is as follows:

"The SLEP data supports the assertion that many drug products can be extended past the original expiration date. . . ."

As a result of all these findings, the federal government has changed its stance on expiration dates. During a recent flu epidemic, a 5-year extension was issued for the use of expired Tamiflu, a drug used to prevent and treat swine flu and other influenzas.

The effective life of a drug usually is in inverse relation to the temperature at which it is stored. In other words, a drug stored at 50 degrees will last longer than one stored at 90 degrees. Freezing, however, affects many drugs negatively. Storing in opaque or "smoky" containers is preferable to clear containers. Humidity will also affect medications, and could even cause mold and mildew to form, especially on natural remedies, such as dried herbs and powders.

Planning ahead, we must consider all alternatives in the effort to stay healthy in hard times. Don't ignore any option that can help you achieve that goal, even expired medicine. We encourage everyone to conduct their own study into the truth about expiration dates; come to your own conclusions after studying the facts.

EMERGENCY CONTACTS

Doctor: _____

Dentist: _____

Fire Dept.: _____

Police: _____

Group Medic: _____

Group Members: _____

_____

_____

_____

_____

_____

_____

_____

_____

_____

_____

_____

_____

_____

_____

_____

GLOSSARY

ABRASION: area of skin scraped off down to the dermis

ABSCESS: collection of pus and inflamed tissue

ACID REFLUX: pain and burning caused by stomach acid traveling up the esophagus

ADRENALINE: name for epinephrine outside the US

AIRWAY: breathing passage

ALLERGY: exaggerated physical reaction to a substance

AMNIOTIC FLUID: liquid inside the pregnant uterus

AMBU-BAG: CPR breathing unit (brand name)

ANAEROBE: organism that doesn't require oxygen to survive

ANALGESIA: pain relief

ANAPHYLAXIS: hypersensitivity to a substance due to antibodies after an initial exposure

ANAPHYLACTIC SHOCK: life-threatening organ failure as a result of hypersensitivity to a substance

ANGINA: heart pain caused by lack of oxygen

ANTIBIOTIC: substances that kill bacteria in living tissue

ANTIBODY: substances produced by the body that respond to toxins

ANTICOAGULANT:	substances that stop clotting
ANTIEMETIC:	substances that stop vomiting
ANTIHISTAMINE:	drugs that relieve minor allergies
ANTI-INFLAMMATORY:	substances that limit inflammation
ANTISEPTIC:	anything that limits the spread of germs on living surfaces
ANTIVENIN:	substance that inactivates snake or insect venom
ANTIVIRAL:	substances that kill viruses
APPENDICITIS:	inflammation of the appendix
ARTERY:	blood vessel that carries oxygen to the tissues
ARTHRITIS:	inflammation of the joints
ASCITES:	fluid accumulation in the abdomen
ASPHYXIANT:	substance that deprives the body of oxygen
ASPIRATION:	inhalation of fluids into the airways
ASTHMA:	shortness of breath caused by a narrowing of airways, often due to an allergic reaction
ASYMPTOMATIC:	without signs or symptoms
ATHEROSCLEROSIS:	blockage of the coronary arteries
AVULSION:	tissue torn off by trauma
BAG VALVE MASK:	CPR breathing apparatus
BANDAGE:	wound covering
BETADINE:	iodine antiseptic solution
BILE:	fluid found in the gall bladder

B.R.A.T. DIET:	diet used to treat dehydration consisting of bananas, rice, applesauce and dry toast
BRONCHITIS:	inflammation of the airways
BRONCHUS:	main respiratory airway
BRUISE:	injury that does not break the skin but causes bleeding due to damaged blood vessels
CAPILLARY:	tiny blood vessel that connects arteries to veins throughout the body
CARDIAC:	relating to the heart
CARTILAGE:	fibrous connective tissue found in various parts of the body, such as the joints, outer ear, and larynx
CATARACT:	a clouding of the lens of the eye
CELLULITIS:	inflammation of soft tissues
CHIN-LIFT:	CPR technique that improves airflow
CHOLECYSTITIS:	inflammation of the gall bladder
CHOLELITHIASIS:	gall stones
CIRRHOSIS:	chronic liver damage
CLOSED FRACTURE:	broken bone that does not break the skin
COLLAPSE SITUATION:	circumstance where modern medical care no longer exists for the long term
COLOSTRUM:	early breast milk rich in antibodies
CONCUSSION:	loss of consciousness caused by trauma to the cranium

CONJUNCTIVITIS: inflammation of the eye membrane

CORNEA: clear covering over the iris

COSTOCHONDRITIS: chest pain caused by inflammation of the rib joints

COTYLEDONS: segments of the placenta

CPR: cardio-pulmonary resuscitation

CROWNING: late stage of labor when the baby's head starts to emerge from the vagina

CURETTAGE: scraping dead pregnancy tissue from the uterus after a miscarriage

CYANOSIS: blue color caused by lack of oxygen

DEBRIDEMENT: removal of dead tissue from a wound

DEHYDRATION: loss of body water content

DERMATITIS: inflammation of the skin

DERMIS: deep layer of the skin

DIABETES: disease in which the body fails to produce enough insulin to control blood sugar levels (type 1) or is resistant to the insulin it produces (type 2)

DIAGNOSIS: identification of a medical condition

DILATION: the act of making more open

DISCHARGE: drainage from a surface or wound

DISINFECTANT: substance that kills germs on non-living surfaces

DISLOCATION: traumatic movement of a bone out of its joint

DISTAL: away from the torso

DIURETIC: substance that increases urine flow

DRESSING: wound covering

DRUG OF CHOICE: best drug for a particular illness

DUODENUM: part of the bowel after the stomach

DYSENTERY: dangerous diarrheal disease

ECLAMPSIA: seizures caused by elevated blood pressures during a pregnancy

ECTOPIC PREGNANCY: pregnancy that implants outside of the womb

EDEMA: fluid accumulation

ELAPID: family of venomous "coral" snakes

ELECTROLYTES: elements found in body fluids

ENDEMIC: native to an area or species

EPIDERMIS: superficial layer of the skin

EPILEPSY: convulsive disorder

EPINEPHRINE: hormone used to treat severe allergic reactions (known as adrenaline outside the US)

EPISTAXIS: bleeding from the nose

ERYTHEMA: redness due to inflammation

ESOPHAGUS: tube that runs from the back of the mouth to the stomach

ESSENTIAL OILS: highly concentrated liquids of various mixtures of natural compounds obtained from plants

EXPECTORANT: substance that loosens congestion

FRACTURE:	a broken bone
FROSTBITE:	frozen tissue, usually in extremities
GALL BLADDER:	organ near the liver that stores bile
GANGRENE:	death of tissue due to lack of circulation
GASTROENTERITIS:	inflammation of the stomach/intestine
GINGIVITIS:	inflammation of the gums
GLAND:	organ that produces hormones
GLUCOSE:	blood sugar
GRAND MAL SEIZURE:	generalized convulsion in epileptics
GRANULOMA:	nodule formed by immune system's attempt to wall off an infection or a foreign object
HEARTBURN:	chest pain caused by stomach acid
HEAT STROKE:	symptoms caused by overheating
HEIMLICH MANEUVER:	action taken to remove foreign object from the airways
HEMOGLOBIN:	red blood cell component that carries oxygen to the tissues
HEMORRHAGE:	blood loss
HEMORRHOID:	varicose vein near the anus
HEMOPTYSIS:	coughing up blood
HEMOSTATIC AGENT:	substance that stops bleeding
HEPATITIS:	inflammation of the liver
HERNIA:	weakness in the body wall
HESITANCY:	difficulty starting a urine stream

HISTAMINES:	substances formed in allergies that cause physical symptoms
HIVES:	bumpy red rash caused by allergies
HORMONE:	substance produced by a gland that affects body functions
HYDRATION:	addition of water to the system
HYGIENE:	cleanliness as health strategy
HYPEROPIA:	farsightedness
HYPERTENSION:	high blood pressure
HYPERTHERMIA:	heat stroke or heat exhaustion
HYPERTHYROIDISM:	condition caused by high thyroid levels
HYPHEMA:	bleeding into the white of the eye
HYPOGLYCEMIA:	low blood glucose levels
HYPOTHERMIA:	syndrome caused by heat loss
HYPOTHYROIDISM:	condition caused by low thyroid levels
IMMOBILIZATION:	prevention of movement
IMMUNITY:	protection against a disease
IMPETIGO:	skin infection with weeping sores
INFARCTION:	death of heart tissue due to lack of oxygen
INFLAMMATION:	reaction to injury characterized by redness, swelling, discharge, pain and heat
INFLUENZA:	viral respiratory illness
INTEGRATED CARE:	treatment using different medical methods

INTOXICATION:	state of being poisoned
INTRAVENOUS:	inside the vein
IRIS:	colored portion of the eye
IRRIGATION:	forceful application of fluid to a wound to clean out debris, blood clots, and dead tissue
IRRITANT:	substance that causes inflammation of tissue
ISCHEMIC:	lacking oxygen due to circulatory failure
JAUNDICE:	yellowing of the skin and eyes due to liver malfunction
KETOACIDOSIS:	life-threatening condition related to failure of blood glucose control
KILOGRAM:	2.2 pounds
LACERATION:	penetration of both skin layers by injury
LARYNX:	the voice box
LASIK:	laser surgery to correct vision
LETHARGY:	extreme fatigue or drowsiness
LIGAMENT:	supportive tissue that connects bones
LITER:	0.264 gallons
LOCALIZED:	isolated to an area
LYMPHATICS:	drainage system for body fluids
MASS CASUALTY INCIDENT:	more victims than available help

MENINGITIS:	inflammation of the brain/spinal cord
MENSTRUATION:	periodic blood flow from the uterus
MIGRAINE:	headaches caused by vascular spasms
MISCARRIAGE:	early pregnancy loss
MOLESKIN:	protective material for blisters
MYOPIA:	nearsightedness
NEUROLOGIC:	pertaining to the nervous system
OPEN FRACTURE:	broken bone that pierces the skin
OPTHALMOSCOPE:	instrument used to look into the eyes
OTITIS:	inflammation of the ear
OTOSCOPE:	instrument used to look into ear canal
OVARY:	female organ that produces eggs
PALPATION:	to feel with the hands
PALPITATIONS:	sensation of dread caused by a rapid heart rate
PATHOGEN:	something that causes disease
PEDIATRIC:	pertaining to children
PELVIC:	pertaining to the bones that provide support for legs and spine
PEPTIC:	relating to stomach acid
PERCUSSION:	to tap on the body to identify hollow and solid areas; for example, when searching for a tumor
PERINEUM:	area between the vagina and anus

PERIOSTEUM:	outside lining of the bone
PETIT MAL SEIZURE:	epilepsy characterized by loss of awareness without generalized convulsive behavior
PHARYNX:	the throat
PHLEBITIS:	inflammation seen in varicose veins
PHLEGM:	mucus discharge from the respiratory tract
PIT VIPER:	snake in the rattlesnake family
PNEUMONIA:	an infection of the lungs
PNEUMOTHORAX:	free air in the lung cavity affecting breathing
POST-ICTAL STATE:	semiconscious state after experiencing a grand mal seizure
POTABLE:	safe to drink
PRE-ECLAMPSIA:	pregnancy-induced hypertension
PRESSURE POINTS:	areas where pressure on blood vessels stops bleeding to distal areas
PROGNOSIS:	likely outcome of a medical condition
PRONE:	lying face down
PROPHYLAXIS:	preventative measures
PROTOZOA:	microscopic organisms that sometimes act as parasites
PROXIMAL:	closer to the torso
PULMONARY:	relating to the lungs
PRURITIS:	itchiness
PULMONARY:	relating to the lungs

PUS: inflammatory discharge caused by the body's response to infection

PYELONEPHRITIS: inflammation of the kidney

QUADRANT: body area divided into quarters

REBOUND: pain elicited by pressing, then made worse by releasing the pressure on a part of the body

REFLUX: acid traveling up the esophagus

RELAPSE: recurrence of a disease's symptoms

RENAL: relating to the kidneys

RESPIRATORY: relating to breathing

RHYTHM METHOD: method of determining fertile periods by tracking menstrual cycles

SALINE: salt water solution used for IV fluids and irrigating wounds

SEBORRHEA: oily, itchy rash on scalp and face

SEDATION: to relax or put to sleep

SEIZURE: convulsion

SHOCK: life-threatening syndrome caused by multiple organ failure or malfunction

SOFT TISSUE: muscle, tendons, ligaments, skin, fat

SPRAIN: damage to a ligament caused by hyperextension

SPHYGNOMANOMETER: instrument used to measure pressure

STERILE: free of germs

STERNUM: breastbone

STETHOSCOPE:	instrument used for listening to heart, lungs, and for evaluating blood pressure
STRAIN:	damage to a muscle or tendon
STROKE:	brain hemorrhage with paralysis
SUBCUTANEOUS:	under the skin
SUPINE:	lying face up
SUSPENSION:	a drug mixed in a liquid
SUTURE:	wound closure with needle and thread
SYNDROME:	collection of symptoms
SYSTEMIC:	condition affecting the entire body
TACHYCARDIA:	elevated heart rate
TENDON:	connection of a muscle to a bone
THERMOREGULATORY:	related to body temperature
TINCTURE:	plant extract made by soaking herbs in a liquid (such as water, alcohol, or vinegar) for a specified length of time, then straining and discarding the plant material
TINNITUS:	ringing in the ears
TOURNIQUET:	item that uses pressure to stop bleeding from a wound
TRAUMA:	injury caused by impact
TRIAGE:	to sort by priority
TUMOR:	a growth in or on the body
TYMPANIC MEMBRANE:	eardrum

ULCER: damage to the wall of the skin, stomach or intestine due to pressure, acid or disease

ULTRAVIOLET: invisible light waves that damage skin or eyes

UMBILICAL: relating to the "belly button"

URGENCY: sudden desire to urinate

URTICARIA: allergic rash

UTERUS: womb

VARICES: enlarged and dilated veins

VASCULAR: relating to blood vessels

VEIN: blood vessel that carries de-oxygenated blood back to the lungs

VERTIGO: dizziness

WHEEZING: high-pitched noises heard while breathing during an asthma attack

INDEX